Food and Drink in Archaeology 2
University of Nottingham Postgraduate Conference 2008

Food and Drink in Archaeology 2

University of Nottingham Postgraduate Conference 2008

Edited by
Sera Baker, Annie Gray, Kay Lakin,
Richard Madgwick, Kristopher Poole
and Michela Sandias

Series Editors: Naomi Sykes and Claire Newton

Prospect Books
2009

First published in Great Britain in 2009 by Prospect Books, Allaleigh House, Blackawton, Totnes, Devon, TQ9 7DL.

© 2009 as a collection Prospect Books.
© 2009 in individual articles rests with the authors.

The authors assert their moral right to be identified as authors in accordance with the Copyright, Designs & Patents Act 1988. No part of this publication may be reproduced, stored in a retrieval system or transmitted in any form or by any means, electronic, mechanical, photocopying, recording or otherwise, without the prior permission of the copyright holders.

ISBN 978-1-903018-68-2

The illustration on the cover is of samian ware, courtesy of the University of Nottingham Archaeology Museum.

For more information about Prospect Books: www.prospectbooks.co.uk.

Design and typesetting in Gill Sans and Adobe Garamond by Tom Jaine.
Printed and bound in Great Britain by The Cromwell Press Group, Trowbridge.

Contents

List of Figures	7
Preface *Sera Baker*	9
Fish Knives, Silver Spoons and Red Dishes *H.E.M. Cool*	11
Irish Names in a London Cemetery: Is it Possible to Identify Irish Immigration in Nineteenth-Century Lukin Street? *Julia Beaumont*	21
Re-enactment and Ritual Consumption: The *Kykeon* in Ancient Mystery Cults *Kirsten Bedigan*	29
The Dun Cow and the Durham Ox: From Dairy to Beef in Eighteenth-Century North-East England *Louisa Gidney*	38
'A Moveable Feast': Negotiating Gender at the Middle-Class Tea-Table in Eighteenth- and Nineteenth-Century England *Annie Gray*	46
The Economic, Social and Environmental Implications of Faunal Remains from the Bronze Age Copper Mines at Great Orme, North Wales *Sian James*	57
An Isotopic Approach to Diet in Medieval Spain *Michelle Mundee*	64
The Ritualization of Eating and Drinking: Politics, Religion and Food Consumption in Pre-Roman Veneto, Italy *Elisa Perego*	73
Infant Feeding and Weaning Practices as Data for Fertility Estimates of a Roman-Period Population Sample from Kellis 2, Dakhleh Oasis, Egypt *Jennifer Sharman*	81
Stable Isotope Analysis of DISH and Diet *Rosa Spencer*	90

Agricultural Crop Choices and Social Change in the Yellow River Valley,
    North Central China during the Late Neolithic and Early Bronze Age   100
Alison Weisskopf

Shorter Contributions

The Dynamics of Fish Consumption in Saxon England   110
Rebecca Reynolds

A Poor Man's Silver? The Role of Pewter in Roman Britain:
    A Collection in the British Museum   117
Lindsey Smith

Eat, Drink and Influence People: The Cutlers' Company Annual Feast   122
Joan Unwin

List of Figures

3.1	The inscription from the false-necked amphora, Eleusis	32
3.2	Man carrying a drinking cup/jug and female with covered vessel on her head participating in the rituals at Eleusis	32
4.1	Examples of the two sizes of cattle bones found at Alnwick	39
4.2	Dun Cow sculpture group on Durham Cathedral	40
4.3	The Durham Ox, detail of painting by Boultbee	40
5.1	J. van Aken: *An English Family at Tea* (c.1720)	49
5.2	Teabowl, c.1820s	51
5.3	Middle-class afternoon tea	53
6.1	General view of the Great Orme Copper Mine, Llandudno	57
6.2	Bone tools from the Great Orme Copper Mine, Llandudno	60
6.3	Comparative graph representing cattle skeletal fragments for Ross Island and Great Orme Mines	61
7.1	Map of Spain	65
7.2	Scatter plot of $\delta^{13}C$ and $\delta^{15}N$ values for Christians from Jaca in comparison with the mean for Muslims in Zaragoza	68
9.1	Kellis 2 cemetery: excavated portion	83
10.1	Skeletons with and without DISH	94
10.2	Males with and without DISH	94
11.1	Map of China	100
11.2	Charts of crop husk phytoliths, and rice leaf/stem versus husk	104
12.1	Digested unidentifiable fish vertebrae	113
12.2	Relative frequencies of herring, cod, whiting, flatfish and eel	114
13.1	Distribution map of pewter small finds, vessels and hoards	118
13.2	Pewter plate bearing the (hidden) Chi-Rho symbol	119

14.1	Page from the accounts of Thomas Moulson, Master Cutler, 1854	123
14.2	The Cutlers' Feast of Mark Firth, Master Cutler, 1867	124
14.3	Menu for the Feast of Charles Belk, Master Cutler, 1885	125

Preface

Building on the success of our 2007 conference, the 2008 Food and Drink in Archaeology conference was held on the 11 and 12 April, again at the University of Nottingham. Unlike the previous year, it was organised in collaboration with archaeology students from three other universities: Cardiff, Reading and York. Papers and posters were structured around four themes. The first, Material Cultures of Consumption, was opened by our keynote speaker, Dr Hilary Cool, whose thought-provoking paper is reproduced in this volume. This session was followed by Scientific Approaches to Food and Drink, Pollution and Purity and finally Dynamics of Foodways. All of the sessions are represented in this volume, which contains a mixture of eleven papers, that were presented orally at the conference, and three shorter articles derived from posters.

Scientific research makes perhaps the greatest contribution, with several chapters presenting the results of isotopic analyses of human remains (see Beaumont, Mundee, Sharman and Spencer). But this is not to suggest that the contents are restricted, far from it. Readers will be introduced to research concerning a wide range of locations and periods, some distant (e.g. Weisskopf's study of archaeobotanical evidence from Neolithic China), while others are more familiar – for instance, Gidney's examination of cattle in eighteenth-century England. And what could be closer to modern British society than 'fish on a Friday' (Reynolds), or more homely than a cup of tea (Gray)? Several of the papers follow Cool in challenging us to move beyond purely functional interpretations – Smith and Unwin's papers demonstrate that plates and bowls can have a far greater significance than being simply middlemen on a food's journey from kitchen to mouth. The idea that food, drink and dining paraphernalia are incorporated into expressions of identity and ideology is reinforced by the work of Bedigan and Perego, both studies examining the more ritualized side of consumption, a theme to which we will return in 2009.

A primary aim of the series has been to provide a platform for post-graduate research and to help develop the skills of research students. All of those involved in the organisation and publication of this conference have benefited greatly from the process. We have been fortunate to be supported by a large number of people. Without the very generous financial support of the Arts and Humanities Research Council (who granted us a collaborative training award) and the University of Nottingham's School of Humanities (who awarded us Roberts' Money) it would not have been possible to run the conference so successfully or publish the proceedings. As important is the scholastic support provided by the many anonymous reviewers who went to such efforts to provide invaluable feedback and advice ensuring the quality of this publication – thank you on behalf of the organizing committee and the contributors.

Sera Baker,
University of Nottingham

Fish Knives, Silver Spoons and Red Dishes

H. E. M. Cool

How can we unlock the past? How can we, as archaeologists, make the communities we explore by excavating their living spaces come alive in all their complexity? I have long thought that one of the best ways to do this is to explore their eating habits, for this is an activity with tendrils that spread into corners of life far beyond the mere ingestion of sufficient calories to keep body and soul together. Fortunately, the remains of food and drink and all the paraphernalia that surrounds its transport, preparation and consumption make up a very large part of the archaeological record. All we need to do is ask these data the right questions, but how do we go about formulating them?

For a start, I suggest it would be helpful if we spent a little time looking at all the paraphernalia surrounding our own consumption patterns and ask, 'What associations does this have, what stories does this tell, what does it say about me?' It is a good training exercise. If you do it, you rapidly realize that artefacts work on many levels other than the prosaically functional. As an example, I'll take three cases of cutlery that sit in one of the drawers of my own kitchen. All three are slender boxes with lids lined with white satin and bases with velvet-covered divisions in which the implements nestle. The small square black one contains six silver teaspoons. A larger and more battered blue case with a broken catch has six small bone-handled steel knives. The largest, black with fancier gilt clasps, has six pairs of bone-handled fish knives and forks with nickel-silvered steel blades. If by some mischance my kitchen was destroyed but the debris were recovered by archaeologists centuries hence, I would expect whoever was researching the site to be able to tell that these utensils were about 70 years old at the time of the destruction. I would expect them to note that they appeared to be sets, whereas the rest of the cutlery in the kitchen is a mismatched jumble. I would hope they would note the spatial separation of the two different categories, for the cases are stored in a different place than the rest of the cutlery. The range of different metals in the sets ought to give them pause for thought. If the cases survived they might note that probably the small knives had seen more wear, given the battered state of their case and the broken catch.

If the small-find specialist dealing with cutlery chatted with the pot specialist, it might dawn on them they had something similar there. A set of six cups, saucers and small plates together with a small bowl and jug all decorated in the same way and in the same very fine fabric (bone china). Again older than the rest of the pottery recovered, retaining all its original members compared to the other sets which have missing members, and spatially separated; though not found with, or even close to, the sets of cutlery. At this point they have a great deal of data on which to start formulating hypotheses. Clearly my kitchen had contained 'special deposits'. I would hope they would realize these were storage rather than use deposits, and that they would make the link between the small size of the knives, spoons and plates and realize that these were likely to have been used together. If they were worth their salt as specialists, they would realize that within the overall kitchen assemblage, this subset of items were candidates for having what Kopytoff (1986) has called a cultural biography. That is to say, something that has been taken out of a life of being an ordinary economic commodity, singularized and set apart. At that point the specialists would need to bring into play their knowledge of the material culture from a period 70 years before the date of the kitchen destruction, to see if they could work out whether these sets would have been unusual in any way when they were new. They could also look at what function the various items fulfilled. Would any of them have been obsolete by the time of the destruction? Why had these items seen such prolonged curation? They might conclude that they were heirlooms, which indeed they are. Entrusted to me for safe keeping when my mother moved to a smaller flat. So what do they say about our family? If I was one of those future specialists, I would start with the fish knives as these would probably be marked down as the most obsolete of the items.

Fish knives are strange. They are deliberately blunt, which seems a contradiction in terms. They were a creation of the Victorian era, as is so much specialist cutlery. How did they come to be part of the goods of the Cool household? This is an interesting question as the Cool household was a place where, on the whole, fish never came. Fish fingers came if you were poorly. Fish and chips came occasionally as a great treat; brought in from outside wrapped in newspaper and placed in the oven to keep warm. Fish as recognizable fish only really came in the form of an occasional smoked haddock fillet to be poached in milk and butter and eaten with toast. For none of these fish occasions were the fish knives and forks thought appropriate. They stayed quietly in their case. They would only have been thought appropriate for proper fish, but in our household that was perceived as dangerous, wild food full of bones.

To understand the Cool-household fish knives and forks you have to divest yourself of all ideas that the material culture surrounding eating and drinking is purely utilitarian, and it will also help to consider the genesis of the type, spurred on as it was by considerations of what things tasted like, technological innovation and changes in society.

In the eighteenth century fish was felt to have too delicate a taste to cope with the taint of the steel cutlery then available. So, for those who could afford it, fish would be traditionally divided up by a silver fish-carver. The development of electro-plating in the nineteenth century did away with the taint of steel and gave the appearance and effect of silver without the cost. As Mrs Beeton said in 1861,

> Where silver fish-carvers are considered too dear to be brought, good electro-plated ones answer very well, and are inexpensive. The prices set down for them by Messers Slack of the Strand are a guinea upward (Beeton 1861, 116).

Fish Knives, Silver Spoons and Red Dishes

Who were these people who could afford fish-carvers at a guinea, and ultimately sets of silver-plated fish knives and forks? Money can best be thought of by seeing what incomes were. That year a charity for distressed clergy and their wives felt that £75 was an adequate annual income to keep a vicar's widow in respectable retirement (Website 1). Mrs Beeton herself noted that an income of £300 would allow a family to have a maid of all work and a nursemaid; you needed £500 a year to afford a cook, housemaid and nursemaid. That guinea would be a large part of the widow's income. It would not be a negligible part of the £300, and for Mrs Beeton's household on £150–200 per annum who could only afford a maid of all work and a girl occasionally, there would be no guineas for fripperies such as these. So in the mid nineteenth century fish knives were for the comfortable middle classes.

By 1940 when the Cool-household fish knives and forks were acquired, they were obviously something that could be aspired to by people much lower down the income scale. My parents belonged to the upper echelons of the southern urban working class. My mother had aspirations for a nice house and it is into that scenario that the unused fish knives and fork fit. It is also of course, the scenario that was to be so cruelly mocked by John Betjeman a decade or so later in his poem *How to get on in society* which uses fish knives in the first line to signify inappropriate pretensions. That poem has the regular refrain that the speaker must have things daintily served, and that certainly sums up my mother's attitude to the presentation of afternoon tea, the meal to which other people were regularly invited. For those the contents of the other two cases, the tea knives and teaspoons, were brought out to join a bone china tea-set on one of her carefully embroidered table cloths with its matching napkins. Within our milieu, preferring afternoon tea to the more substantial high tea was, of course, another sign of social aspiration (Davidson 1999, 6, 380–1).

So these 'special deposits' in my kitchen had been singularized because they were artefacts that played a very active role in the way in which an individual presented herself to the world. The ritual of Sunday afternoon tea was one that structured my youth. Each Sunday we would be either entertaining or being entertained by friends and family, it was the way bonds were forged and maintained. The tea things were a conspicuous part of this but the fact that we had the fish knives and forks safe in their case, in the unlikely event we should ever entertain people to a meal including fish, was also important for the household's self-image, even if not so conspicuous.

A background like this is a good training ground for the type of artefact specialist I am. I didn't need to read works of theory that told me that objects had cultural biographies, I knew from childhood that all things have their stories. In the case of the silver spoons it would be recited regularly: who had given them and in what circumstances. The challenge we face as archaeologists is to reconstruct those stories and what they tell us about the people using them. To realize that it is the context that gives meaning, not the artefact itself; and that the physical context in which it is found (pit or layer) is only the starting point for the definition of that context. My mother's fish knives say aspiration. The ones I use at Da Fiori say 'we are part of the restrained dining experience at the best restaurant in Venice, we are one of the things that qualify it for its Michelin star'. Da Fiori's fish knives are confident and much used. My mother's were aspirational and anxious, and much preferred staying in their case.

Why use a spoon?

Roman Britain is the place where I spend most of my time and it is a very data-rich area. The sites are generally well dug, all the modern techniques of finds retrieval are normal, and a great deal of money is spent on specialist reports. To make the best use of this wealth, we need considerably more integration of data than is normal at present. The same could be said of most other periods and areas of archaeological investigation. If we do start to integrate the data, can we push the boundaries of what artefacts signified to those who used them in the way I have explored the cutlery in my kitchen? As an example let us stay with cutlery and examine the role of spoons in early Roman Britain. This is an interesting period, as the formal incorporation of Britain into the Roman Empire was accompanied by a whole variety of new practices and their accompanying artefacts, spoons being one of them.

Some years ago I explored to what extent native Britons were prepared to accept the change to their eating habits implied by the adoption of the spoon (Cool 2004a, 28–30). The typical spoon of the first to second centuries is the very distinctive round-bowled *cochleare* which was made in a range of materials suitable for all pockets, and so not just restricted to the richer elements of society. There is always the problem we face of whether just because an artefact looks familiar, it was used in what to us would be the appropriate way. In this case, as discussed in the original paper, there are grounds for thinking the spoons were used for eating. By comparing the incidence of spoons to that of hair pins, another new introduction made in a wide range of materials, it was possible to show that they became increasingly less common the further down the settlement hierarchy one went. It seems reasonable to conclude that away from the more cosmopolitan urban centres, the native population were rejecting new modes of eating whilst at the same time the women were very happy to adopt new hairstyles. Having established this basic pattern, can we use it to explore further?

By good chance we can if we start looking at certain burials in the south-east/south central area of England. In that area there is a cremation burial tradition that spans the later first to mid second century and which is contemporary with the use of the *cochleare*. The graves are often found as isolated examples or as pairs. Probably the most spectacular were those found at Bartlow on the Essex/Cambridgeshire border in the 1830s, where the deceased were buried under barrows. Unfortunately many of these burials were either found as antiquarian finds or more recently by metal detectorists and so the quality of the information is often not as high as one would wish for, but much can still be done with them (for references see Cool 2006, 193–9).

Fish Knives, Silver Spoons and Red Dishes

A regular feature of these graves are multiple sets of vessels for eating and drinking, but there are also various other types of artefacts that suggest the deceased were being placed in the grave with suites of material that was explicitly thought to be 'Roman'. At Bartlow, for example, the barrows variously include a folding iron chair of the type used by magistrates, a regular combination of a metal jug and basin of the types used in sacrifice for washing hands, strigils and oil flasks for visits to the baths. The location of the burials in rural sites or outside the lesser *civitas* capitals is such as to strongly suggest these are the burials of a native elite, and the grave goods suggest they are coming to terms with what it was to lead an elite life within the Roman empire, i.e. what it meant to be Roman. They are explicitly things for leading a Roman life: a magistrate's chair, the correct vessels for sacrifice, the correct accoutrements for going to the baths, the correct equipment for showing you are literate. Sets of bright red pots are also a feature, the deceased normally went to the grave with several place settings as if company would be expected in the afterlife. So what was their understanding of the correct way to eat?

It is useful to examine one found at Winchester in some detail (Biddle 1967, 230–45). It was a rescue excavation caused by the exposure of a corner of the grave in a sewer trench in 1964. It was conducted under less than ideal conditions and, given its date, no environmental sampling is to be expected, as that is a more recent development of archaeological practice. Despite the drawbacks, most of the deliberate positioning of all the elements could be ascertained and conclusions drawn from them.

A large shale tray had been placed in the grave and on it were a large pottery bowl, pork bones with associated knives and a round-bowled spoon. To one side there was a group of three pottery cups, a glass jug and a copper-alloy jug. Beyond them was a group of small items which, from their distribution, were probably originally deposited in a bag. These included items such as gaming counters, melon beads, a little bell and the pretty part of seal box. There was another group of vessels at the other end of the grave. This consisted of pottery cups and dishes as well as a flagon and jar. At least one of the dishes had probably also contained food, given that it was covered by a second inverted dish. With this group of vessels there was a stylus and wax-smoother used in writing.

Within this grave there were two groups of items that can immediately be seen to be falling into the 'what it was to be Roman' category. These are the writing equipment and group of cups and jugs – the latter indicating that the deceased was expected to consume their wine with water in the approved Roman way. The presence of pork might also fall into this category, as it was not generally part of the everyday diet of native Britons, though it was a regular part of a contemporary Italian diet (Cool 2006, 82–4 for discussion; see also King 1999). It is necessary to be somewhat cautious of this interpretation, as the pork might represent an earlier Iron Age tradition. In Dorset, just to the south-west of the area where this grave was found, pork joints were felt to be appropriate for the grave, but not for everyday life for some individuals (Maltby 2002, 69). Perhaps in this milieu pork was reserved for the gods. All sorts of taboos can develop around food and it may be that that the other guests expected in the afterlife were deities.

For our current investigation, it is the presence of a spoon that is of most interest. This is one of very few of these graves where a spoon is present. In general, while adopting all sorts of other elements of 'being Roman', the native elite did not appear to embrace the spoon, given both the evidence of the domestic pattern and the contents of these graves themselves. One suspects they would have been uncomfortable at a contemporary Mediterranean dinner party where it was expected one would be using spoons to convey food to the mouth, and where the table would be equipped with a silver table service, such as the one from the house of the Menander at Pompeii, where spoons feature prominently (Painter 2001). Expressing *romanitas* through other aspects of life was acceptable; using spoons to convey food to the mouth was a change too far. So what is different about the individual buried in this grave?

It is useful at this point to look at who was being buried. The osteologist said the cremated remains suggested immaturity (perhaps a teenager) or a slender female. The excavator decided on the basis of the drinking equipment, the gaming counters and writing equipment that this was a man's grave; but that probably says more about the excavator's preconceptions of what was appropriate for each sex than it does about the inhabitant. Probably of more use is to look at the group of equipment which contained the unfeminine gaming counters. Bells nearly always indicate young people when they are found in Roman graves, as the young seem in special need of the protection that *tintabulum* can bring (Cool 2004b, 401). The group as a whole is very reminiscent of the *crepundia* (things that jangle) that were often placed in the graves of girls who had died before they could be married (Martin-Kilchner 2000). If that is correct, then that group represents another aspect of exploring what it was to be Roman, as depositing *crepundia* does not appear to be a native British habit. On balance therefore, I think we are more likely to be looking at a female teenager than a male one. It is an intriguing thought that the spoon may have been acceptable here because it was women who may have been at the forefront of adopting new consumption habits and the accoutrements that went with them.

What we have done in this little exploration is to move from a broad-brush approach to establish the general pattern that initially native Britons did not generally adopt spoons. We then found another set of data to explore it further (the general pattern in the graves) and then picked up an anomaly and looked to see why it should be there. To be able to do the latter we had to be able to spot that the graves were expressing a particular take on what it was like to be native elite within a new world order, to understand what messages some of the grave goods were sending out, and to spot that the little bag of goodies said 'female', which might give us an explanation. Quite a lot of these things are nothing explicitly to do with eating and drinking but they demonstrate the framework within which we need to work, if we want to explore the topic.

Before we can make progress, we do have to consider the methodological barriers that lie before us. Modern archaeology has fragmented into many different specialisms. This is understandable given the sheer volume of data and the very different skills needed to explore different aspects of it. We must be careful not to work simply within our own little areas. We must all work at integrating the data much more than is often the case, and to be able to do this needs some basic data standards. We must keep in mind that the ultimate aim is to illuminate the lives of the people who lived in the past, not to provide *comparanda* for our fellows who work in the same area as we do. Always the fundamental need is to present the data in such a way that they can easily be interrogated and used in systematic intra- and inter-site comparisons. For this there must be rigorous standards for quantification. I have written extensively on this topic elsewhere (see for example Cool 2006, 9–11), and do not propose to explore it in detail here; but it cannot be stressed too often that assemblage comparisons across a variety of sites allow basic patterns of consumption to be established and that without the underpinning of rigorous quantification you cannot get them. Unless you can quantify a category of find in a way that will give consistent results when faced by similar groups elsewhere, you can make little progress. Quantification is not a sexy topic: it is like typology – tedious but vital. It forms, however, the foundations on which we can erect our stories of the past and as we all know, any edifice without firm foundations is likely to be somewhat insecure. But once we have those virtuous foundations, what stories we can tell using eating and drinking practices as the window on the past. Quite often a very different sort of place emerges from that found in standard texts.

The north-south divide

In my own area of Roman Britain there is a great deal that is written on the difference between the north and the south. Yet there is one difference that would have been immediately apparent to anyone who lived at that time and who travelled from north to south or vice versa, and it virtually never gets considered. That difference comes from the different staples that the regions preferred. In the south the standard grain was spelt wheat, in the north it was barley. We can tell this from carbonized grains that the environmentalists so carefully retrieve and report on (for references see Cool 2006, 77). There was no real environmental reason for this, spelt could have been and was grown in the north, but most people there preferred barley. When these grains are thought of not as cereal but as the products they were made into, the implications of this are immediately apparent.

With spelt wheat you can make a risen loaf, it has the right sort of insoluble proteins that will form gluten and it is the gluten that allows the dough to form the open texture of a risen loaf. Barley, by contrast, does not have these proteins. There is no point in attempting to make risen bread from it, but it does make good griddle cakes. These can be equally tasty but are distinctly flatter.

The other main use of grain in the Roman period was to brew beer. We can tell what sort of grain was being used because the malting processes sometimes went wrong, leaving us with charred grain which is almost indestructible in the archaeological record. The malted grain deposits in the south are invariably of wheat and so wheat beer was being drunk (see Cool 2006, 141–2). To date I am not aware of any malted grain deposits from the north but one might suspect that it was based on barley. Wheat beer and barley beer are very different drinks both in taste and in appearance. So the south was a land of risen bread and pale beer, the north one of griddle cakes and dark beer. Truly two different places. It is worth pausing for a moment to consider how the communities would have looked at each other. Fundamental differences in the types of foods consumed by neighbouring communities are often seized on by one or the other to reinforce their feelings of innate superiority. We can recall that in the eighteenth century, when England and Scotland were still exploring what it was like to be yoked together in the Union, Dr Johnson was famously dismissive of the Scots via his definition of oats: 'A grain, which in England is generally given to horses, but in Scotland appears to support the people.' One wonders if people coming from the south in Roman Britain experienced the same cultural disdain.

Theoretically, the Romans should certainly have seen the northern British as a lower grade of people, as traditionally in their cultural milieu barley was food for horses and a punishment ration for the army. Yet it is not unusual to find granaries stocked with barley on northern forts and some of this certainly seems to have been for human consumption (see Cool 2006, 77–9 for references). From the dates of these deposits, it seems unlikely that the units were being reduced to living off the land and using barley because that was all that was available. Instead this too may have been the cultural preference of the unit in garrison. In some instances the military units clearly came from the Danubian area and there is no reason why they should have the same prejudices and tastes as a unit from Italy. Just as differences in basic foodstuffs can separate communities, so similarities can give rise to fellow feeling. In Romano-British studies the current fashion is for seeing the military as a community that was separate from the civilian population (see for example Mattingly 2006). One does wonder, judged by the foodstuffs, whether in some areas the dichotomy was quite so strong.

Given that in some academic areas food is still seen as a little beyond the pale and a bit frivolous, I suspect we shall have an uphill battle to convince those who write popular books on Roman Britain that charred grain is a major source of information about how people lived: but it is a battle worth fighting.

Anorexic Christians

So far we have looked at material culture to show how the integration of all these facets with other things we know about the society and the sites they come from can push forward our understanding of eating and drinking practices. In turn, this enhanced knowledge can be used to formulate new questions. One area we have not looked at yet is the evidence of the people themselves as preserved in their skeletons. As can be seen by looking at the evidence from Poundbury, similar approaches to human skeleton remains can yield interesting results.

Knowing what the normal pattern is for the data from a particular environment is vital if you are going to be able to tease out the most from your data. Obviously if you don't know what normal is, then you cannot spot deviation. To some extent Poundbury became the norm for the cemeteries of fourth-century urban populations as it was one of the first cemeteries in Britain to have the bodies subject to full modern osteological analysis, and to be published (Farwell and Molleson 1993). As information from an increasing number of comparable cemeteries has become available, it has started to be apparent that far from being the norm, Poundbury appears distinctly odd. The people were much sicklier than many comparable populations, the bodies showed a much higher incidences both of dental caries, and of the skeletal changes that show stress in childhood (summarized Cool 2006, 24–6). There is a lot of evidence that the people were not eating properly. There was, too, an over-representation in the cemetery of girls who had died between their late childhood and early adulthood, that is, who had died early. Why was this? The osteologist could offer no explanation other than to say it must reflect the way girls were treated from a young age.

Again, integration of all the elements might offer further light. This is one of the few cemeteries of a population in Roman Britain which can be identified with some degree of certainty as having Christian elements – given that a painted mausoleum helpfully included a Chi Rho (Hartley *et al* 2006, 207, no. 193 fig. 37). Fasting to the point of anorexia seemed to be something that many of the early Church fathers advocated for females (Grimm 1996, 170–1). Could this be what the unusually high death rate amongst young females is reflecting here? It seems a distinct possibility. The extent to which Christianity was, or was not, practised in the fourth century is again a matter of much debate in the scholarly literature on Roman Britain. What impact this might have had on the daily lives of its practitioners, of the sort we may be seeing here, is very rarely considered. Yet this would imply an adoption of the faith much more profound than the mere wearing of an amulet with a Christian symbol, the sort of evidence much discussion centres on.

Conclusions

So if I had to summon up my key points, what would they be? The answer is simple. Consider the context, think about quantification, integrate your data and avoid compartmentalization. It heartens me that there is so much post-graduate endeavour being poured into the subject of eating and drinking in the past, as evidenced by the conference from which these papers stemmed. When I sent the Cambridge University Press the outline for my book, it wasn't called *Eating and Drinking in Roman Britain*, that was just the sub-title. It was called *Send More Beer* after a writing tablet at Vindolanda which articulates the real concerns of the men at this outpost of empire at the end of the first century (Bowman and Thomas 2003, 84 no. 628). Their main worry was that the beer had run out. The publishers were anxious as to whether a subject so inherently frivolous as eating deserved their imprimatur, and so the title was changed to reassure the reader that the book was suitably weighty and dull enough for an academic press. The amount of work currently being devoted to exploring foodways suggests that it is an area of investigation that is moving to a central position in archaeology. This is an excellent thing, and not just because it means that future authors of books similar to mine will not have disguise them with worthy but deeply boring titles. Brillat Savarin's fourth aphorism is much over-used these days, but as a discipline we have taken too long to embrace the concept of 'tell me what you eat and I will tell you what you are'. It is an approach that can cast an abundance of new light on many dusty corners of the past. We need to embrace all parts of our discipline and work together because it is only through integration of many different strands of information that we will be able to do justice to the complexities of the past.

References

Beeton, I. 1861. *Mrs Beeton's Book of Household Management* (Oxford World's Classics edition 2000).

Biddle, M. 1967. 'Two Flavian burials from Grange Road, Winchester', *Antiquaries Journal* 47, 224–50.

Bowman, A.K. and Thomas, J.D. 2003. *The Vindolanda Writing Tablets (Tabulae Vindolandenses) Volume 3* (London).

Cool, H.E.M. 2004a. 'Some notes on spoons and mortaria', in Croxford, B., Eckardt, H., Meake, J. and Weekes, J. (eds), *TRAC 2003: Proceedings of the Thirteenth Annual Theoretical Roman Archaeology Conference Leicester 200* (Oxford), 28–35.

Cool, H. E.M. 2004b. *The Roman Cemetery at Brougham, Cumbria* (London, Britannia Monograph 21).

Cool, H.E.M. 2006. *Eating and Drinking in Roman Britain* (Cambridge).

Davidson, A. 1999. *The Oxford Companion to Food* (Oxford).

Farwell, D.E. and Molleson, T.I. 1993. *Poundbury Volume 2: the Cemeteries* (Dorchester, Dorset Natural History and Archaeological Society Monograph 11).

Grimm, V.E. 1996. *From Fasting to Feasting: the Evolution of a Sin* (London).

Hartley, E., Hawkes, J., Henig. M. and Mee, F. 2006. *Constantine the Great: York's Roman Emperor* (York)

King, A. 1999. 'Meat diet in the Roman world: a regional inter-site comparison', *Journal of Roman Archaeology* 12, 168–202.

Kopytoff, I. 1986. 'The cultural biography of things', in Appadurai, A. (ed.), *The Social Life of Things* (Cambridge), 64–91.

Maltby, M. 2002. 'Animal bone from graves', in Davies, S.M., Bellamy, P.S., Heaton, M.J. and Woodward, P.J. (eds) *Excavations at Alington Avenue, Fordington, Dorchester, Dorset, 1984–87* (Dorchester, Dorset Natural History and Archaeological Society Monograph 15), 168–70.

Martin-Kilcher, S. 2000. '*Mors immatura* in the Roman world – a mirror of society and tradition', in Pearce, J., Millett, M. and Struck, M. (eds) *Burial, Society and Context in the Roman World* (Oxford), 63–77.

Mattingly, D. 2006. *An Imperial Possession* (London).

Painter, K.S. 2001. *The Insula of the Menander at Pompeii. Volume IV: the Silver Treasure* (Oxford).

Website 1 : http:www.londonancestor.com/charity/pensions/orphan-widow.htm – checked 10 February 2009.

Irish Names in a London Cemetery: Is it Possible to Identify Irish Immigration in Nineteenth-Century Lukin Street?

Julia Beaumont, University of Bradford

The study of population movement has always been central to archaeology, with the appearance of new material cultures (Wilson 1976; Brodie 1997), changes in animal husbandry or plant cultivation (King 1978; 1991; Jones 1991 21–28) and shifts in burial practices (Crawford 1997, 69–70) traditionally being cited as evidence for migration or invasion. Recently, studies of diaspora have undergone a renaissance, largely due to the emergence of new scientific techniques that allow patterns of mobility to be reconstructed from the isotopic systems (Bentley 2006; Larsen 1990). Most of these studies have concentrated on prehistoric populations, but some studies have examined the historic period, combining scientific and artefactual data with documentary evidence to great effect (Cox *et al.* 2001; Miles and Powers 2006; Montgomery *et al.* 2009). Such studies have the potential not only to improve our understanding of a historical period, but also to test the validity of interpretations so that they might be applied to prehistoric periods with greater confidence. With particular reference to a recently-excavated population from Lukin Street cemetery in Whitechapel (London), this chapter will examine the potential of isotope analysis for investigating diet and migration in a period that is perceived as a watershed in Irish history: the Great Famine, or Potato Famine (1847–1848).

The Great Famine: its causes, impact on diet and as an impetus for migration

The Irish Potato Famine (1847–1848) was the culmination of a long period of political and social upheaval that resulted in mass emigration. The scale of the disaster, in which at least a quarter of the population died – the approximate figure of two million being an underestimate (O'Grâda 1999, 87) – was due to a combination of social, economic, demographic and 'natural' factors.

In pre-famine Ireland the population appears to have been relatively healthy, evidenced by its rise from five million to just over eight million between 1780 and 1841 (Swift 2002, 4). According to the census of 1841, most people (66 per cent) were dependant on agriculture but although a variety of food-crops was grown commercially, most of these were exported, leaving potatoes as the chief source of food for the indigenous population: the average Irish male was eating 12–14lb of potatoes per day supplemented only by oatmeal, dairy products, eggs, and fish in coastal populations (Litton 1994,15; O'Neill 1976, 211). Whilst this diet allowed the Irish to achieve a comparatively tall stature – on average 70 inches, compared with 68.5 inches for the English and 68 inches for the Belgians (Davis 1991, 13) – the population was vulnerable when this staple food crop failed, especially since the pattern of employment of the rural farm workers meant that they did not earn cash, and so could not afford to buy alternative sources of food during periods of need (O'Gráda 1999).

When the potato blight reached Ireland in 1845, it coincided with a five-year period of cold winters and wet summers which allowed the fungus to remain in the soil. The most common potato, 'the lumper', grown by the cottiers (labourers) for their own table, was particularly susceptible to the blight. At first, it was felt that the potato crop failure was a one-off, limited to certain areas. When crops failed again the following year a crisis developed, exacerbated by the Corn Laws, which restricted the import of cheap food from abroad, and the prevailing political views on Ireland (e.g. the Malthusian approach – that famine, disease and war were a natural check to rising population), which limited the Government's response to the growing famine (O'Neill 1976, 209f). Early attempts by the government to provide for the destitute relied on the unpopular local workhouses and the provision of work for aid: seemingly pointless projects such as breaking rocks and building roads which went nowhere. The money allocated for these projects was expected to be repaid by the Irish ratepayers, who were themselves often cash-poor (O'Gráda 1999, 50).

There was an attempt made by Sir Robert Peel in 1845–46 to relieve the widespread famine by the importation of maize ('Indian meal') from America. This unfamiliar food was unpopular, difficult to process and cook: its yellow colour and effects on the intestines of the starving locals led to its being renamed 'Peel's Brimstone' (O'Neill 1976, 216). When outdoor relief was eventually provided in the form of dry food, the bureaucratic administration meant that this was subject to fraud, with landlords favouring their tenants, and food being sold rather than reaching those in need (O'Gráda 1999, 70f). Provision of cooked food in order to avoid such abuse meant that families had to travel to the distribution centres, often long distances, at a time when they needed to conserve calories (O'Gráda 1999, 71). Contemporary sources describe a starving population who left their homes to go to areas where they hoped to receive food and medical help (Litton 1994, 95f). These nutrition-depleted individuals were particularly susceptible to infectious diseases such as the lice-borne typhus and yellow fever. The doctors and clergy who worked with the destitute also suffered high levels of disease and many died as a result (MacArthur 1976, 279). There are descriptions of starving and swollen individuals that are consistent with the protein deficiency disorder kwashiorkor described in the African famines of the twentieth century (Shetty 2006) and with vitamin B deficiency, known as *beriberi*. In some areas the death rate was so high that eye-witness accounts describe people buried at the roadside where they died, or in their dwellings as burial grounds were overwhelmed (MacHugh 1976, 419f).

The severity of the famine varied across Ireland. Some districts, particularly the north and east, were less reliant on the rural economy and could afford to buy alternative foods: the populations of Munster and Connaught were twice as likely to die as those of Ulster and Leinster (O'Grâda 1999). In the south and west, the Catholic, Gaelic-speaking cottiers left their homes to avoid destitution, death or eviction, and clearances were common (Swift 2002, 6). Those landlords with resources often assisted their tenants in leaving the district. Some paid for their tenants' passage from Ireland (MacDonagh 1976, 332f). The emigrants tended to follow particular routes when leaving Ireland; whilst those with the resources would travel via English ports to the Americas or Australasia, the poorest would remain in England or Scotland. Those travelling to London are most likely to have come from the south and west, via Cork and Bristol (Swift 2002, 27) and may be from the area which experienced the worst deprivation. There is evidence that Irish surnames found in the epigraphic records of cemetery populations (Miles and Powers 2006), some of which can be traced to particular districts, may also be a guide to the origins of the individual or their parent (Website 1).

Irish emigration

There was already a well-established pattern of seasonal migrant workers, and step-wise emigration to America, Canada and Australasia via English ports: at the end of the Napoleonic war in 1815, the settlement of Irish-born soldiers in England was just a part of the estimated 50,000 emigrants per year (Swift 2002, 3). The recording of the actual number leaving Ireland is probably inaccurate and complex. The population of Ireland peaked at over 8 million in 1841 (Swift 2002, 54), in spite of the considerable number of people who chose to leave Ireland to live abroad in search of a better life. The prevailing culture of 'exile' (Swift 2002, 7) from their homeland meant that some migrants eventually returned home when their economic circumstances permitted. Some were forcibly repatriated from other areas of Britain when they were deemed to be destitute (Swift 2002, 74). What is clear is that the famine caused a huge rise in the number of people leaving Ireland: approximately one million people left between 1815 and 1845. A peak of at least one and a half million was reached between 1845 and 1851; from 1851 to 1914, a further four million emigrated (Swift 2002, 3).

At least one quarter of all Irish emigrants settled in Britain: records for 1851 show that over a quarter of a million people left Ireland with approximately 108,000 finally settling in London, some via other cities such as Bristol. Their eventual destination was often determined by their ports of departure and arrival, by family connections in the town or city and by the availability of suitable work, whether skilled or unskilled. Many joined the already-established Irish community in London where, by 1851, 4.6 per cent of the population were Irish-born (Swift 2002, 35). By 1897, 24 per cent of the population of Whitechapel were immigrants (Powers 2008).

Arriving in London – a new diet

Contemporary accounts of the food eaten by the poor in London suggest that this was dramatically different to that of south-west Ireland. Londoners in the mid-nineteenth century had access to a range of foods – both local and imported via the Thames, by road and later by rail – limited only by ability to pay (Tames 2003, 31).

Until the new railway system was established and could carry perishable food into the capital quickly enough to arrive at the markets in a fresh state, most of the residents ate locally-produced vegetables. The wealthy could and did indulge in imported treats (Pickard 2005, 192; Tames 2003, 100f) but the most exotic import enjoyed regularly by the lower classes was tea (Tames 2003, 79). Sainsbury's became one of the first importers of milk via rail, and fish was imported to Billingsgate market from the east-coast ports from the 1850s onwards (Tames 2003, 79). However, it is important to remember that wheat for the bread, the staple of the labourer, may have been grown in Ireland or elsewhere in the Union, although not imported from further afield because of the Corn Laws (O'Neill 1976, 210).

White (2007, 132) describes the living conditions of Whitechapel and its Irish population during the pre-famine era: 14,000 Irish Catholics lived in six riverside parishes near the docks in 1816. In that year, for example, '700 Irish and 100 pigs' were living in a narrow court of twenty-four small houses. It appears that livestock was kept throughout the city, with cows providing milk from back yards and even cellars (Pickard 2005, 30). Fruits and vegetables sold in the many markets in the capital were generally grown in market gardens, initially within the city, and from 1796 until the 1880s in Barking to the east, as far as Ealing in the west by 1800, and along the south bank of the Thames (Tames 2003, 81f).

W.B. Tegetmeier's *Manual of Domestic Economy* (1858) contains suggestions for his middle-class female readers, who might be visiting the poor with an eye to improving or supplementing their diet, that have some bearing on the situation in earlier decades (Pickard 2005, 180). A labourer's daily intake should include 2lb of bread and two pints of milk. He suggests keeping a pig if possible, and lists the cheapest cuts of meat with cooking instructions (boiling rather than roasting and using bones for broth). Fish could be had cheaply at close of day at Billingsgate (those visiting the poor describe their dwellings as smelling overwhelmingly of fish). Mayhew (1985, 16, 66) describes onions, 'sparrow grass' (asparagus) and watercress as common additions to the diet. Those in domestic service were often given part of their wages as 'beer and tea money' (Pickard 2005, 149). Often people would drink weak ale as an alternative to the unpleasant local water (Pickard 2005, 149), and tea was a luxury. Small and larger breweries were plentiful in the city (White 2007, 173) and also used the local water.

Thus far it is possible to piece together a generalized picture of the diet that confronted the Irish immigrants on their arrival in London. However, archaeology and, in particular, stable isotope analysis of human remains have the potential to check the validity of this picture and consider migration and diet at the level of the individual.

The potential of isotope analysis and Lukin Street cemetery, Whitechapel

Isotope analysis of human remains has been successfully used to construct dietary histories (Ambrose 1993; Larsen 1990; Sealy 2001) and examine migration patterns in ancient populations (Sealy *et al.* 1995; Montgomery *et al.* 2005). In post-medieval cemeteries, cultural groups can potentially be identified by the examination of evidence such as artefacts, name plates, funerary practices and osteological analysis (Cox *et al.* 2001; Miles and Powers 2006; Powers 2008). However, without supporting documentary evidence, this is still open to interpretation. The Catholic cemetery at Lukin Street presents an opportunity to combine archaeological and osteological evidence with historical evidence concerning individuals' likely origins, religious practices, education, health, housing and occupations. By using these data as a framework it may be possible to investigate the validity of isotopic indicators of both migration and diet, as carried out in the study of the Cape Town underclass by Cox *et al.* (2001).

The Lukin Street cemetery was consecrated as the cemetery of the Catholic Mission of St Mary and St Michael, and was in use for just 11 years (1843–1854), so contains the remains of individuals who died before, during and after the famine of 1847–1851. In 2005 the cemetery was partially excavated by the Museum of London Archaeological Service (MoLAS), recovering samples of 747 individuals. Of these, 194 have partially legible coffin plates which indicate that 32 of the 49 recorded surnames are of Irish origin, some from specific regions of Ireland; this may reflect expatriate communities that already existed in this area, as well as recent immigrants. In addition, two of the nameplates are thought to be of Spanish and Portuguese individuals (Miles and Powers 2006; Powers 2008). As such, the cemetery provides the opportunity to obtain an isotopic profile for a temporally-constrained population, some of whom are likely to have survived and escaped from the Great Irish Famine (Miles and Powers 2006).

Currently, samples of human hair, cortical bone, tooth dentine and tooth enamel are being taken for stable isotope analysis. These different tissues turn over at different rates and so will reflect an individual's diet at different stages during their life. For instance, dental enamel and dentine do not remodel once formed and therefore the isotopic signatures provided by teeth will reflect diet during childhood and early adulthood (the age at which different teeth develop is well known – see Hillson 1996). By contrast, bone remodels throughout life and, for older individuals, bone of different densities may reflect the dietary intake at different times of life (Bell *et al.* 2001). The analysis of bone apatite and collagen gives information about different dietary components (Ambrose *et al.* 1997). Scalp hair grows at approximately 1.5 cm per month and thus contains information about the diet in the weeks and months just prior to death (Wilson and Gilbert 2007). By studying a range of these different skeletal elements in the Lukin Street population, it is expected that four main dietary regimes may be identifiable from carbon and nitrogen isotope ratios. These regimes may be characterized as follows:

1) a diet containing meat, fish and mainly C_3 plants consumed by those living in London. This varied diet, available even to the poor of the East End (Tames 2003,

193), should be identifiably different, in terms of isotope ratios, from that of Irish immigrants.

2) the restricted pre-1847 (C_3) potato diet eaten by the rural Irish poor which may resemble a vegetarian diet, indeed similar to local herbivores, and which can be distinguished from the diet of a true London omnivore.

3) a diet of almost exclusively (C_4) maize eaten by those receiving Sir Robert Peel's imported famine relief (O'Neill 1976, 212f). Maize (a C_4 plant) metabolizes carbon in a way that produces in the human body different isotope ratios to those plants (C_3 plants) which were being eaten in Ireland at the time of the famine. Larsen *et al.* (1990) used both carbon and nitrogen isotopes to distinguish between marine-based diets and C_4 diets.

4) the nutritionally-stressed famine diet when little or no calories are consumed. It is likely that individuals subject to the harshest conditions, the most limited range of foods and the onset of dietary deprivation, would show the most marked effects on the stable isotope ratios of their skeletal remains. Mekota *et al.* (2006) showed how body mass index was related to changes in the nitrogen isotopes of individuals deliberately depriving themselves of food.

The analysis of other isotope systems would also be useful in confirming migration of individuals with unusual dietary signatures. The isotope ratios of oxygen (Fricke *et al.* 1995) and radiogenic elements in tooth enamel such as strontium and lead (Montgomery *et al.* 2005; Haverkort *et al.* 2009) have been shown to vary depending upon place of residence, climate and ingested food and drink, and may be used as independent evidence of migration for those individuals with an unusual, non-local dietary signature.

By analysing a range of different isotopes from a combination of tissue-types, life histories for individuals and the wider population can be compiled and these can then be related to known historical records of famine and migration in the mid-nineteenth century.

Conclusions

When attempting to identify migration within a post-medieval burial ground, it is possible not only to use the evidence found during the excavation, but also the available historical and documentary evidence about the site, the surrounding district and the potential places of origin of migrants. The evidence available from records of the time indicates that there are very likely to be survivors of the Irish famine buried in the cemetery at Lukin Street.

The four potential dietary regimes which could be identified from carbon and nitrogen isotope analysis of the skeletal remains are: the varied London diet, the pre-famine potato diet, the high maize relief diet, and the starvation stage of the famine. Hair keratin, bone and dentine collagen will provide isotope ratios correlated to those of the foods ingested at the time of tissue formation. Therefore, the measured isotope ratios can represent different times of life. Some individuals may have lived through two or more of these regimes.

Investigation of the skeletal tissues may help distinguish between populations who have grown up with very different diets, and migration may be then be confirmed using oxygen and radiogenic isotopes such as strontium and lead in the tooth enamel. The combination of the results of isotope analyses with the available osteological, funerary and documentary evidence should identify first-generation Irish immigrants buried in the cemetery at Lukin Street and add to the knowledge about the effects of dietary stress on the skeletal tissues.

Acknowledgements

I would like to thank the following for their help in this study: Natasha Powers, Don Walker and the team at MoLAS, and Janet Montgomery, Julia Lee-Thorp, Chris Knüsel, Andy Wilson, Andy Gledhill and Victoria Mueller at the University of Bradford.

Bibliography

Ambrose, S.H. 1993. 'Isotopic analysis of paleodiets: methodological and interpretive considerations', in Sandford, M.K. (ed.) *Investigations of Ancient Human Tissue. Chemical Analyses in Anthropology* (Langhorne, PA.), 59–130.

Ambrose, S.H., Butler, B.M., Hanson, D.B., Hunter-Anderson R.L. and Krueger H.W. 1997 'Stable isotope analysis of human diet in the Marianas archipelago, Western Pacific', *American Journal of Physical Anthropology* **104**, 343–61.

Bell, L.S., Cox, G. and Sealy, J. 2001. 'Determining isotopic life history trajectories using bone density fractionation and stable isotope measurements: a new approach', *American Journal of Physical Anthropology* **116**, 66–79.

Bentley, R.A. 2006. 'Strontium isotopes from the earth to the archaeological skeleton: Review', *Journal of Archaeological Method and Theory* 1–53.

Brodie, N. 1997. 'New perspectives on the Bell-beaker Culture', *Oxford Journal of Archaeology* **16**, 297–314.

Cox, G., Sealy, J., Schrire, C. and Morris, A. 2001. 'Stable carbon and nitrogen analyses of the underclass at the colonial Cape of Good Hope in the eighteenth and nineteenth centuries', *World Archaeology* **33**, 73–97.

Crawford, S. 1997. 'Britons, Anglo-Saxons and the Germanic Burial Ritual', in Chapman, J. and Hamerow, H. (eds) *Migration and Invasions in Archaeological Explanation* (Archaeopress), 45–72.

Davis, G. 1991. *The Irish in Britain 1815–1914* (Dublin).

Fricke, H.C., O'Neil, J.R. and Lynnerup, N. 1995. 'Oxygen isotope composition of human tooth enamel from medieval Greenland: linking climate and society', *Geology* **23**, 869–72.

Haverkort, C.M., Weber, A., Katzenberg, M.A., Goriunova O.I., Simonetti, A. and Creaser, R. A. 2009. 'Hunter-gatherer mobility strategies and resource use based on strontium isotope (87Sr/86Sr) analysis: a case study from Middle Holocene Lake Baikal, Siberia' *Journal of Archaeological Science* **35**, 1265–80.

Hillson, S. 1996. *Dental Anthropology* (Cambridge).

Jones, M. 1991. 'Food production and consumption-plants' in Jones, R. (ed.) *Britain in the Roman Period: Recent Trends* (Sheffield), 21–28.

King, A. 1978. 'A comparative survey of bone assemblages from Roman Britain', *Bulletin of the Institute of Archaeology* **15**, 207–32.

King, A. 1991. 'Food production and consumption – meat', in Jones, R. (ed.) *Britain in the Roman Period: Recent Trends* (Sheffield), 15–20.

Larsen, C.S. 1990. *The Archaeology of Mission Santa Catalina de Guale: 2. Biocultural Interpretations of a Population in Transition* (New York).

Litton, H. 1994. *The Irish Famine: An Illustrated History* (Dublin).

MacArthur, W.P. 1976. 'Medical history of the famine', in Edwards, R.D. and Williams, T.D. (eds) *The Great Famine: Studies in Irish History 1845–52* (New York), 263–315.

MacDonagh, O. 1976. 'Irish emigration to the United States of America and the British colonies during the famine', in Edwards, R.D. and Williams, T.D. (eds) *The Great Famine: Studies in Irish History 1845–52* (New York), 319–388.

MacHugh, R.J. 1976. 'The famine in Irish oral tradition', in Edwards, R.D. and Williams, T.D. (eds) *The Great Famine: Studies in Irish History 1845–52* (New York), 391–435.

Mayhew, H. 1985. *London Labour and the London Poor* (London).

Mekota, A., Grupe, G. Uger, S. and Cuntz, U. 2006. 'Serial analysis of stable nitrogen and carbon isotopes in hair: monitoring starvation and recovery phases of patients suffering from anorexia nervosa', *Rapid Communications in Mass Spectrometry* **20**, 1604–10.

Miles, A. and Powers, N. 2006. *Bishop Challoner catholic collegiate school, Lukin Street, London, E1: a migration in post-medieval London post-excavation assessment and updated project design* (unpublished report MoLAS, London).

Montgomery, J., Evans, J.A., Powlesland, D. and Roberts, C.A. 2005. 'Continuity or colonisation in Anglo-Saxon England? Isotope evidence for mobility, subsistence practice and status at West Heslerton', *American Journal of Physical Anthropology* **126**, 123–38.

Montgomery, J., Muldner, G. and Cook, G. 2009. 'Isotope analysis of bone collagen and tooth enamel', in *"Clothing for the Soul Divine" Burials at the Tomb of St Ninian. Excavations at Whithorn Priory, 1957–67* (Edinburgh).

O'Grâda, C. 1999. *Black '47 and Beyond: The Great Irish Famine in History, Economy and Memory* (Princeton).

O'Neill, T. 1976. 'The organisation and administration of relief, 1845–52', in Edwards, R.D. and Williams, T.D. (eds) *The Great Famine: Studies in Irish History 1845–52* (New York), 209–254.

Pickard, L. 2005. *Victorian London* (London).

Powers, N. 2008. '"All the outward tinsel which distinguishes man from man will have then vanished…" an assessment of the value of Post-Medieval human remains to migration studies', in Brickley, M. and Smith, M. (eds) *Proceedings of the Eighth Annual Conference of the British Association for Biological Anthropology and Osteoarchaeology* (Oxford), 41–49.

Sealy, J., Armstrong, R. and Schrire, C. 1995. 'Beyond lifetime averages: tracing life histories through isotopic analysis of different calcified tissues from archaeological human skeletons', *Antiquity* **69**, 290–300.

Sealy, J. 2001. 'Body tissue chemistry and palaeodiet', in Brothwell, D.R. and Pollard, A.M. (eds) *Handbook of Archaeological Sciences* (Chichester), 269–80.

Shetty, P. 2006. 'Malnutrition and undernutrition', *Medicine* **34**, 524–9.

Swift, R. 2002. *Irish Migrants in Britain 1815–1914: A Documentary History* (Cork).

Tames, R. 2003. *Feeding London – A Taste of History* (London).

White, J. 2007. *London in the Nineteenth Century "A Human Awful Wonder of God"* (London).

Wilson, D.M., 1976. 'Scandinavian settlement in the north and west of the British Isles: an archaeological point of view' *Transactions of the Royal Historical Society*, Fifth Series **26**, 95–113.

Wilson, A.S. and M.T.P. Gilbert, 2007. 'Hair and nail', in Thompson, T. and Black, S. (eds) *Forensic Human Identification* (Boca Raton), 147–74.

Website 1: www.censusfinder.com – consulted 22 April 2008.

Re-enactment and Ritual Consumption: The *Kykeon* in Ancient Mystery Cults

Kirsten Bedigan, University of Glasgow

Ancient and modern sources agree that *kykeon*, a barley-based concoction, played a fundamental role in ritualistic practices in antiquity, both spiritual and secular. In the Eleusinian mysteries it appeared to be integral to the initiatory practices of the cult, which are strongly connected to re-enactments performed by the initiates. These traditions seem to be grounded in the use of *kykeon* as a traditional gesture of hospitality. This paper briefly discusses the various functions of *kykeon* and its relationship to ritual before examining its role in the Eleusinian mysteries in more detail, from its part in the initiatory practices to the symbolic nature of the ingredients. This model of *kykeon* and initiation is then discussed in relation to the mystery cults of Isis and the Kabeiroi, whose rituals appear to mimic those of the Eleusis.

	Sources	Barley	Water	Wine	Milk	Honey	Mint & Herbs	Onion	Drugs	Egg	Goat's Cheese
1	*Homeric Hymn to Demeter*, lines 198–211	•	•				•				
2	Homer, *Iliad*, 11.624	•		•		•		•			•
3	Homer, *Odyssey*, 10.290, 316	•		•		•			•		•
4	Modern Recipe, Dalby and Grainger 2000, 41	•	•			•				•	•
5	Hippocrates' Recipe, Norrie 2003, 26	•		•	•						
6	Hippocrates' Recipe, King 1998, 121	•	•								

Table 3.1. Ingredients for ancient and modern recipes for kykeon.

The *kykeon* in the ancient sources

Both spiritual and secular, the *kykeon* played a key role in ritual practice. Its nature could change according to the function required, and these variations depended heavily on the different ingredients incorporated into the recipes and the context in which it was used (Table 3.1). There appear to have been three main functions: 1) as a remedy in a medicinal or palliative sense, 2) as a standard gesture of hospitality, and 3) as an integral part of ritual activities (Rosen 1987, 425).

1) Remedy (Table 3.1, Nos. 5–6)

That *kykeon* was offered as a solution to, or a remedy against, illness is apparent in the medicinal writing of Hippocrates and Galen (Craik 1995, 392; Delatte 1955, 28–30; Rosen 1987, 417). As a medical remedy, it was suitable for certain problems like consumption, enlargement of vessels in the lungs, and fever in otherwise healthy patients – see Hippocrates *Internal Affections* (trans. Potter 1988, 4 and 12) and *Diseases II* (trans. Potter 1988, 43); King 1998, 121 and Norrie 2003, 26 – but not others such as an ulcerated trachea or 'acute' diseases, i.e. high fevers (Craik 1995, 392 and see Hippocrates *Regimen for Acute Diseases* (trans. Potter 1988, 39)). The question of it as a means of relief is harder to explain. It can be identified as a drink which relieved poverty, hunger and misery (Delatte 1955, 27; Rosen 1987, 417, 421). There is no justifiable explanation for this, although it may be linked to the myth presented by the anonymous *Homeric Hymn to Demeter* (trans. Cashford and Richardson 2003, 197–200) which related the story of the abduction of Persephone, Demeter's mourning for the loss of her daughter and the establishment of the Eleusinian cult. Its association with ritual, specifically mourning, may represent a transition from a liminal phase to that of an aggregative stage (laughter and joy, breaking of the fast) (Bell 1997, 94; Lincoln 1979, 230); this may relate to initiation into the cult of Demeter and Persephone.

2) Hospitality (Table 3.1, Nos. 1–3)

Kykeon was portrayed as the drink of hospitality offered by Nestor in Homer's *Iliad* (trans. Murray 1924, 11.624–41) (Delatte 1955, 24–25). Here it was a refreshing beverage, a quality not normally associated with a barley-based pottage, especially one containing goats' cheese and onion. Evidence from other literary sources confirms the thirst-quenching properties of the *kykeon* (Ovid *Metamorphoses*, trans. Raeburn 2004, 5.448–54).

In contrast with the hospitality of Nestor in the *Iliad*, the manner in which Circe prepared and used *kykeon* in the *Odyssey* (trans. Murray 1924, 10.234–35) was a perversion of good host-guest relations (Delatte 1955, 25). Circe's *kykeon* enchanted the crew of Odysseus and ultimately transformed them into swine. The *kykeon* she created was practically identical to Nestor's and would at face value suggest that the basic recipe was harmless. It is only through the addition of drugs that the nature of the concoction is altered.

3) Ritual (Table 3.1, No. 1)
   Perhaps like the remedial function of *kykeon*, the ritual connotations of the drink derived from the *Homeric Hymn to Demeter* (trans. Cashford and Richardson 2003, 198–211). In this context the *kykeon*, as a foodstuff, has a clear and definite role in initiation into the cult of Demeter and Persephone at Eleusis (Delatte 1955, 30; Gooch 1993, 10; Iles Johnston 2003, 170). In many ways *kykeon* was a symbolic representation of the desire to be initiated (Rosen 1987, 424), and this can be demonstrated by the iconography. At the Villa of the Mysteries at Pompeii, a scene depicts a group of satyrs, one of whom is peering closely into a bowl. This figure, because of the intensity of his gaze, is sometimes argued to be looking at or in the act of receiving a bowl of *kykeon* (Mudie Cook 1913, 167, pl.11). Although this cannot be positively ascertained, it does at least firmly place the concept of *kykeon* in a strongly ritual context.

The *kykeon* in the mysteries of Demeter and Persephone

The sanctuary of Demeter and Persephone at Eleusis was the only sanctuary where the use of *kykeon* in the rituals can be confirmed. There is no definitive evidence that *kykeon* was used at other sanctuaries (Fotopoulos 2003, 87), although there are similarities which can be identified such as the manner in which the ceremony was conducted and the vessels used (Delatte 1955, 13). It is clear, however, that there were differing attitudes regarding consumption within the cult which help explain the variations in ritual practice. Some sanctuaries, Eleusis included, prohibited wine, whereas others (for example Corinth) had no such restrictions (Bookidis 1987, 481).

As part of the initiation the *dromena*, or re-enactment, took place within the Telesterion at the sanctuary at Eleusis (Preka-Alexandri 2000, 20–21). The exact nature of the *dromena* is unclear, but it would appear that the focus was placed on the abduction of Persephone, along with the display of sacred objects (Preka-Alexandri 2000, 21). It is presumed the *kykeon* was incorporated into this stage of the initiation (Mylonas 1947, 143). Its ritual use is to some extent confirmed by Demeter's statement in the *Homeric Hymn to Demeter*, that she will consume the *kykeon* 'for the sake of the rite' (trans. Cashford and Richardson 2003, 212). Further information can be retrieved from Clement of Alexandria's description of the password known to Eleusinian initiates, 'I fasted, I drank the *kykeon*, I took from a chest, I did something, I put into a basket and from a basket into a chest' (*Exhortation to the Greeks*, trans. Butterworth 1919, 21.2). Clinton (1992, 35 n.107) disagrees with this interpretation, refuting the presence of *kykeon* in the actual initiation. This alternative proposal argues that *kykeon* was part of the rites of the *Thesmophoria* and not the Eleusinian Mysteries, and that Clement conflated the activities from the two cults (Clinton 1992, 35 n.107). However, Clinton's comments on the idea that *kykeon* was eminently suitable for ritual cast doubts upon his dismissal of the potion from Eleusinian initiation (*ibid.*).

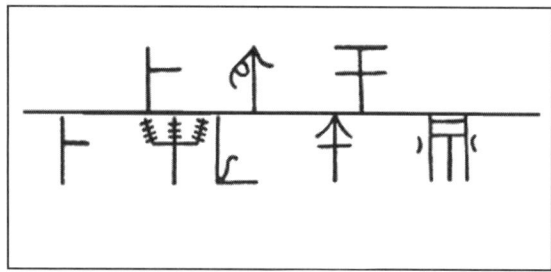

Figure 3.1. The inscription from the false-necked amphora, Eleusis (after Mylonas 1936, 428 fig.16).

The mourning nature of Demeter's (and the initiates') fast and the subsequent consumption of the *kykeon* as a transitional stage can be seen in some of the archaeological evidence from the sanctuary. A false-necked amphora (*c*.1200 BC), excavated from the area of a Late Helladic III structure, carries an intriguing inscription (see Figure 3.1 and Mylonas 1936, 426; 1947, 135). If we accept Mylonas' transcription of symbols, based on the premise that they are read right to left; the text reads '*pa-i-da | ku-ka-o-ne-da*', 'Oh maiden, this potion here' (Mylonas 1936, 429); however, Forbes (1949, 356–57) is critical of this translation since Mycenaean texts are read left to right. There are two possible meanings: firstly, that the potion was a dedication or libation to Persephone (the maiden); the initiate consumed the *kykeon* as part of a process of mourning for the lost Persephone. Secondly, that the initiate received the potion from or on behalf of Persephone (Mylonas 1936, 429). Both interpretations demonstrate the commemorative nature of the *kykeon*, which is an aspect previously noted by some scholars (Lord 1967, 246).

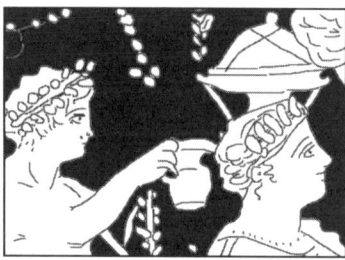

Figure 3.2. Man carrying a drinking cup/jug and female with covered vessel on her head participating in the rituals at Eleusis, from the Ninnion tablet (after Preka-Alexandri 2000, 17 fig.9).

The *kykeon* vessels, for both mixing and serving, can be seen on the Ninnion tablet (Figure 3.2). Two female figures are shown with lidded vessels upon their heads; this was believed to be the container for *kykeon* (Kerényi 1967, 181–82). Elsewhere in the scene, a male figure is shown carrying a small jug or drinking cup, supporting the idea that the *kykeon* was consumed en-route to the sanctuary (Kerényi 1967, 178–79; Storey 2003, 166–67). However, the presence of Demeter and Persephone within the depiction would suggest that the *kykeon* has been prepared and brought to the sanctuary for the ritual, a theory which will be discussed later in further detail.

The case for purposeful barrenness

In the *Homeric Hymn to Demeter*, Demeter's choice of herb flavouring in the *Homeric Hymn* is interesting (trans. Cashford and Richardson 2003, 209). The mint used is γλήχων, an Ionic form of βλήχων, pennyroyal (*Mentha pulegium*). Pennyroyal has many medicinal functions, including use as an abortifacient (Delatte 1955, 39; Riddle 1991, 18). The knowledge of the properties of the plant would presumably have been well known, as Aristophanes was able to make jokes about the herb in many of his works which played on the idea that the plant was a contraceptive. One of the main references to this is in *Peace* (trans. Hall and Geldart 1907, 706–12) where the Boeotian lady in the scene is complimented on her trim figure, which contrasts with the supposedly visible pregnancies of the other characters; the implication is that she is fully aware of the use of abortifacients. Others, however, assert that pennyroyal was associated with birth and nursing (Clinton 1992, 35 n.107), a not anomalous function in an agricultural- and fertility-focused cult. Further evidence indicates that this herb was also used as a wine flavouring (Andrews 1958, 148).

On learning of her daughter's abduction, Demeter refused to let anything grow on earth (Fotopoulos 2003, 71). Her consumption of a known oral contraceptive is almost a symbolic reference to the current state of the earth. Her role as goddess of agriculture has such strong connotations that it seems difficult to reconcile the premise of a fertility deity consuming contraceptives. This had to be a deliberate act on the part of Demeter, or more likely, the author of the hymn, to emphasize the barren situation.

Since the *kykeon* was consumed by initiates we have to conclude that the quantities of pennyroyal included in the potion were very low. We could also presume that the amounts involved were in keeping with the herb's use as a wine flavouring (Andrews 1958, 148), rather than at a level of a medicinal dosage. Given that there are no reports of abortion or other events amongst pregnant initiates, it would seem unlikely that the dosage was high enough to induce miscarriage (Dean-Jones 1994, 143). This implies that the inclusion of pennyroyal was symbolic of barrenness and infertility rather than as a functional abortifacient.

Exploring the potential psychoactive elements

Although the basic recipes provided for the *kykeon* give no hint of anything that could be described as intoxicative (Rosen 1987, 423), it seems unlikely that it was simply a harmless substance. The prohibition of wine at the sanctuary may indicate that something else was added to the recipe (Bookidis 1987, 481; Delatte 1955, 31). Studies from elsewhere in the world certainly suggest that specific plants or compounds could have been used as additives to provide a psychotropic aspect to religious rituals (Samorini 1996, 40–41).

Pennyroyal is known to have a narcotic effect (Kerényi 1967, 179), although this is very mild (Watkins 1978, 15). It is possible that the recipe provided in the *Homeric Hymn* is inaccurate, either purposefully or accidentally, and that pennyroyal is used as a cover for another, more powerful ingredient.

Other studies suggest that ergot, a form of fungus growing on barley and other grasses, was a part of the mixture used at Eleusis (Luck 2001, 137). As a fungal strain, it bears similarities with other psychoactive compounds and would certainly be capable of inducing hallucinations. Part of the problem with accepting the idea of ergotism derives from the scepticism voiced in previous studies (Luck 2001, 135). Burkert (1987, 108) is dismissive of the concept on the basis of the substance's (allegedly unpleasant) effects and the problems of ensuring an adequate annual supply. It was unlikely that such compounds would be used unless supplies were consistent and maintainable (Burkert 1987, 108), but this cannot be confirmed. The major objection, that ingesting ergot had negative effects, does cast doubts on the use of the fungus within this ritual. Since initiation at Eleusis was meant to be a positive event, it would seem unlikely that ergot was a popular or even sensible choice.

Alternatively, it is possible that the mix of barley and water was prepared earlier and allowed to develop into a form of beer (Kerényi 1967, 178–79). Aside from these opinions, evidence for the pre-initiation preparation of *kykeon* is scanty. The major source cited by the majority of scholars as proof that the potion was prepared and consumed before reaching the sanctuary is a fragment from Eupolis' *Demoi* (Storey 2003, 166–67). Here a foreigner, unused to the practices of Eleusis, is portrayed as having barley on his upper lip, implying that he has consumed his *kykeon* too early (Storey 2003, 166). Whilst this provides some interesting evidence that a barley mixture was partaken en-route to the sanctuary, there is no proof that this was actually the *kykeon* used in the Eleusinian mysteries (Storey 2003, 167). This fragment may indeed represent a parody of the mysteries (Delatte 1955, 37). Mylonas' (1961, 259) argument, that the initiates partook of the *kykeon* in the same order of activities as Demeter in the Homeric Hymn, would imply that the potion was prepared and imbibed at the beginning of initiation – a practice leaving no time for fermentation to take place.

The *kykeon* in other cults?

Clinton (1992, 35 n.107) offers the theory that the *kykeon* was a drink appropriate to ritual and that its absence would be peculiar; he proposes that this potion was certainly used in the *Thesmophoria* and possibly also other religious celebrations (see also Delatte 1955, 48, and 56). Beyond Greece, the association between barley and gods was also prevalent. In Egypt, barley was closely linked with religious rituals (Newman and Newman 2006, 5); Isis in particular has strong connections with barley, often being known as the 'lady of bread, of beer' (Witt 1997, 16–17). Merkelbach (1995, 481) refers to the *kykeon* in relation to the cult of Isis and briefly suggests that the meal of bread was a sacred rite on the same level and nature as the Eleusinian mixture. Further similarities between the cults of Demeter and Isis can be seen in the fasting preceding the initiation ceremony (Heyob 1975, 58–59); *kykeon* would be a logical foodstuff with which to break the fast. Even if the use of the *kykeon* cannot be confirmed, there does seem to be a level of theatricality about the cult of Isis. The procession to the sanctuary described in Apuleius' *Metamorphoses* (trans. Hanson 1989, 11.8) includes humans and animals dressed in the guise of figures from mythology.

The relationship between Isis and the Kabeiroi was curious (Witt 1971, 154); the Kabeiroi have associations with agricultural fertility and seafaring which reflect some of Isis' attributes (Price and Kearns 2003, under *Cabiri* and *Isis*). There are sites with evidence of worship of the Kabeiroi which also have associations to Isis and Serapis (Bedigan 2008, 403 no.7, 410 no.25). On the basis of the iconography, the cult of the Kabeiroi at Thebes has strong connections with *kykeon*: several vases from the Theban sanctuary depict Circe and Odysseus with the *kykeon* (Bedigan 2006, 14–15 nos.10–14). From the available evidence relating to initiation into the Kabeiric cult, the ceremony seems to resemble the Eleusinian model quite closely, even if the specifics were different (Lehmann 1998, 37–38). There is no literary evidence to indicate the consumption of *kykeon*, but the choice of iconography is peculiar. The only explanation that can be offered was that the scene was either re-enacted at the Theban sanctuary or that it was directly related to the initiatory procedures.

Conclusion

It cannot be refuted that the *kykeon* was a multi-functional concoction. However, within the ancient texts it was closely bound up with the idea of hospitality. The *kykeon* was offered as the ideal in guest-host relations, whether as an act of good manners in the *Homeric Hymn* and *Iliad,* or in a perverted form in the *Odyssey*, where it is used as means for forced transformation. It is only when mythology becomes entwined with religion that the *kykeon* takes on its ritual function. In the *Homeric Hymn to Demeter*, Demeter's acceptance of the *kykeon* confirms its ritual function at Eleusis (trans. Cashford and Richardson 2003*,* 212). The concept of re-enactment on the part of the initiate is clear. They, like Demeter, fast and break that activity by consuming *kykeon*; at the same time they are mourning the loss of Persephone and also rejoicing in her rise from the underworld. That the Eleusinian mysteries offered salvation after death (Burkert 1987, 21), was surely bound up with this story. In the same way, the idea that *kykeon* gave relief can be connected to the hymn; there is no reason to suppose that the relief offered by the drinking of *kykeon* was granted during life, and it is possible that the gift was provided in the afterlife. Clinton's (1992, 35 n.107) argument that the *kykeon* was used at the *Thesmophoria* and that its alleged use in the Eleusinian mysteries was a misattribution belies his comment elsewhere that the *kykeon* was eminently suitable for all mystery cults. Evidence from Egypt and Greece could certainly be incorporated to support the theory that *kykeon* or a similar substance was used in many different cults and in a similar manner to Eleusis (Merkelbach 1995, 481). The issues relating to the proposed toxicity are interesting, but the more important aspect to consider was the symbolic nature of the *kykeon*. Its very presence identifies the cult as a mystery, and its role within initiation cannot be denied. Whilst it could be drunk in isolation away from ceremonies, it is these rituals which shape the initiate; the re-enactment of relevant myths and stories would provide a fitting setting for such a drink.

References

Andrews, A.C. 1958. 'The mints of the Greeks and Romans and their condimentary uses', *Osiris* 13, 127–49.
Bedigan, K.M. 2006. 'Changed appearances: the use of masks on the ceramics from the Theban Kabeirion in Greece', *eSharp* 8, 1–23.
Bedigan, K.M. 2008. *Boeotian Kabeiric Ware: The Significance of the Ceramic Offerings at the Theban Kabeirion in Boeotia* (Unpublished PhD Thesis, University of Glasgow).
Bell, C. 1997. *Ritual: Perspectives and Dimensions* (Oxford).
Bookidis, N. 1987. 'The sanctuary of Demeter and Kore: an archaeological approach to ancient religion', *American Journal of Archaeology* 91, 480–81.
Burkert, W. 1987: *Ancient Mystery Cults* (Cambridge, Mass.).
Butterworth, G.W. (trans.) 1919. *Clement of Alexandria, Exhortation to the Greeks* (Cambridge, Mass.).
Cashford, J. and Richardson, N. (trans.) 2003. *Homeric Hymn to Demeter* (London).
Clinton, K. 1992. *The Iconography of the Eleusinian Mysteries. The Martin P. Nilsson Lectures on Greek Religion, delivered 19–21 November 1990 at the Swedish Institute at Athens* (Stockholm).
Craik, E. 1995. 'Diet, diatia and dietetics', in Powell, A. (ed.) *The Greek World* (London), 387–402.
Dean-Jones, L. 1994. 'Review of J.M. Riddle, Contraception and Abortion from the Ancient World to the Renaissance (Cambridge, 1992)'. *Journal of the History of Sexuality* 5, 142–144
Delatte, A. 1955. *Le Cycéon, Breuvage Rituel des Mystères d'Éleusis* (Paris).
Forbes, W.T.M. 1949. 'The inscription on the Eleusis vase', *American Journal of Archaeology* 53, 356–7.
Fotopoulos, J. 2003. *Food Offered to Idols in Roman Corinth, A Social-Rhetorical Reconsideration of 1 Corinthians 8:1–11:1* (Tübingen).
Gooch, P.D. 1993. *Dangerous Food: 1 Corinthians 8–10 in its Context* (Waterloo, Ontario).
Hall, F.W. and Geldart W.M. (trans.) 1907. *Aristophanes, Peace* (London).
Hanson, J.A. (trans.) 1989. *Apuleius, Metamorphoses, or The Golden Ass* (Cambridge, Mass.).
Heyob, S.K. 1975. *The Cult of Isis Among Women in the Graeco-Roman World* (Leiden).
Iles Johnston, S. 2003: '"Initiation" in myth, "initiation" in practice: the Homeric Hymn to Hermes and its performative context', in Dodd, D.B. and Faraone C.A. (eds) *Initiation in Ancient Greek Rituals and Narratives: New Critical Perspectives* (London and New York), 155–80.
Kerényi, C. (trans. R. Manheim) 1967. *Eleusis, Archetypal Image of Mother and Daughter* (Princeton).
King, H. 1998. *Hippocrates' Woman: Reading the Female Body in Ancient Greece* (London and New York).
Lehmann, K. 1998. *Samothrace: A Guide to the Excavations and the Museum* (Thessaloniki, 6th Edition).
Lincoln, B. 1979. 'The rape of Persephone: a Greek scenario of women's initiation', *Harvard Theological Review* 72, 223–35.
Lord, M.L. 1967. 'Withdrawal and return: an epic story pattern in the Homeric Hymn to Demeter and the Homeric Hymns', *Classical Journal* 62, 241–8.
Luck, G. 2001. 'Review of R. Gordon Wasson, A. Hofmann and C.A.P. Ruck, The road to Eleusis (Los Angeles, 1998)', *American Journal of Philology* 122, 135–8.

Merkelbach, R. 1995. *Isis Regina – Zeus Sarapis. Die griechisch-aegyptische Religion nach den Quellen dargestellt* (Stuttgart and Leipzig).
Mudie Cook, P.B. 1913. 'The paintings of the Villa Item at Pompeii', *Journal of Roman Studies* 3, 157–74.
Murray, A.T. (trans.) 1919. *Homer, The Odyssey* (London).
Murray, A.T. (trans.) 1924. *Homer, The Iliad* (London).
Mylonas, G.E. 1936. 'Eleusiniaka', *American Journal of Archaeology* 40, 415–31.
Mylonas, G.E. 1947. 'Eleusis and the Eleusinian mysteries', *Classical Journal* 43, 130–46.
Mylonas, G.E. 1961. *Eleusis and the Eleusinian Mysteries* (Princeton).
Newman, C.W. and Newman R.K. 2006. 'A brief history of barley foods', *Cereal Foods World* 51, 4–7.
Norrie, P.A. 2003. 'The history of wine as medicine', in Sandler, M. and Pindar, R. (eds) *Wine: A Scientific Exploration* (New York and London), 21–55.
Potter, P. (trans.) 1988. *Hippocrates, Internal Affections* (Loeb edition vol. VI, Cambridge, Mass.).
Potter, P. (trans.) 1988. *Hippocrates, Diseases 2* (Loeb edition vol. V, Cambridge, Mass.).
Potter, P. (trans.) 1988. *Hippocrates, Regimen in Acute Diseases* (Loeb edition vol. VI, Cambridge, Mass.).
Preka-Alexandri, K. 2000. *Eleusis* (Athens, 3rd Edition).
Price, S. and Kearns, E. 2003. *The Oxford Dictionary of Classical Myth and Religion* (Oxford).
Raeburn, D. (trans.) 2004. *Ovid, Metamorphoses* (London).
Riddle, J.M. 1991. 'Oral contraceptives and early-term abortifacients during classical antiquity and the middle ages', *Past and Present* 132, 3–32.
Rosen, R.M. 1987. 'Hipponax fr.48 Dg. and the Eleusinian *kykeon*', *American Journal of Philology* 108, 416–26.
Samorini, G. 1996. 'An African *kykeon*?', *Eleusis* 4, 40–41.
Storey, I.C. 2003. *Eupolis, Poet of Old Comedy* (Oxford).
Watkins, C. 1978. 'Let us now praise famous grains', *Proceedings of the American Philosophical Society* 122, 9–17.
Witt, R.E. 1971. *Isis in the Graeco-Roman World* (London).
Witt, R.E. 1997. *Isis in the Ancient World* (Baltimore).

The Dun Cow and the Durham Ox: From Dairy to Beef in Eighteenth-Century North-East England

Louisa Gidney,
University of Durham

Among the many innovations and achievements of the later eighteenth century is the phenomenon popularly referred to as the Agricultural Revolution, with people like Turnip Townsend celebrated for popularizing the eponymous vegetable and Bakewell for his impact on principles of livestock breeding. Such programmes of investment were not undertaken without the guarantee of a return, and these changes in basic agricultural production were stimulated by demand from an increasing industrial and urban population. The traditional rural staple of 'white meats' (dairy products), was replaced in the towns by meat, carrying the fat to be used as suet and dripping in the cookery that became associated with coal-fired ranges. It is only recently that the archaeology of this period has been seen as filling out the history written from the viewpoint of educated and wealthy men. The animal bones found in the rubbish dumps of this period round out the story of when, and how fast, changes occurred in the animals kept and, by inference, their produce. Taken in conjunction with artistic representations of cattle and the written sources, this paper will consider the factors involved in the replacement of the local small dairy cattle with the large improved beef cattle from perspectives other than those of the affluent and literate.

The excavation of an evaluation trench at Alnwick Castle, Northumberland (Archaeological Services 2006) revealed a stone-lined pit with one fill deposit producing 41 cattle lower leg bones (seventeen metacarpals and twenty-four metatarsals), with associated pottery dated to between the late eighteenth and early nineteenth centuries. Due to the limited extent of this test excavation, there is no further information on the origin of this deposit.

It was immediately apparent that two distinct phenotypes of cattle were represented in this collection of bones (Figure 4.1). Fewer in number, only five metacarpals and two metatarsals, are bones of the small, indigenous cattle: these particular bones would be visually indistinguishable if placed with either Romano-British or medieval finds of cattle bones from north-east England. Such small, gracile adult bones generally indicate the slaughter of cows. The five smaller metacarpal bones from Alnwick have a greatest length range of 165–192 mm, which overlaps the range of 152–182 mm (N=11) for the modern Dexter cows contained in my reference collection. The other type is very large, with a range of 214–237 mm, and is taken to be physical evidence for the improved Durham Shorthorn associated with the famous livestock breeders of this period, such as the Culley and Colling brothers (Bailey 1810). The presence of some unfused distal epiphyses and clear fusion lines among the larger bones indicate that these animals were younger at slaughter than the small cattle. Only one of the modern Dexters approaches the size of the larger specimens from Alnwick, with a greatest length of 214 mm. This animal was a cross-bred steer castrated as a young calf and not beefed until its fourth year. The distal fusion line is still clear. Heterosis, or hybrid vigour from cross-breeding, and a change in the age of castration may be part of the explanation for the large size of the Alnwick bones.

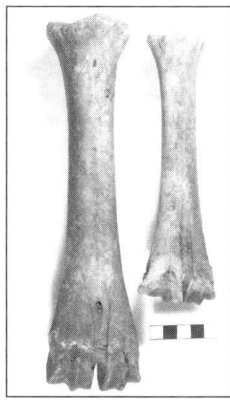

Figure 4.1. Examples of the two sizes of cattle bones found at Alnwick (Jennifer Jones, Archaeological Services Durham University).

The cattle metapodial bones from Alnwick are not unique. Urban finds of the large improved type in the region are also known from Masham (Stokes and Huntley 1998), and the combination of large and small cattle from late eighteenth-century deposits at Whitby (Gidney 2002). Unfortunately these excavations were both assessments, so no metrical data are available for comparison with the Alnwick bones. Rural finds of skeletons of the large animals are known from St Giles by Brompton Bridge (Stallibrass 1993), but are undated. The two skeletons with fused metacarpals fall at the larger end of the Alnwick range with greatest lengths of 227 mm and 239 mm. The Alnwick bones therefore represent a snapshot of a phenomenon represented from Northumberland to north and east Yorkshire.

Two iconic representations of cattle, broadly contemporary with the finds from Alnwick, illustrate examples of these small and large cattle. The Dun Cow sculpture on Durham cathedral, dated post 1780, depicts a small cow (Figure 4.2), while the painting of the Durham Ox by Boultbee, engraved by Whessell and published in 1802 (Comben 2007), portrays a large steer (Figure 4.3).

The sculpture of the Dun Cow on Durham cathedral is of a small cow of dairy type, attended by two milkmaids in late eighteenth-century dress. Although this tableau illustrates part of the founding legend of the cathedral, the depiction of the cow and dairymaids was intended to be understood by eighteenth-century viewers. This cow is a small animal with classic dairy conformation; she has every point noted as an ideal

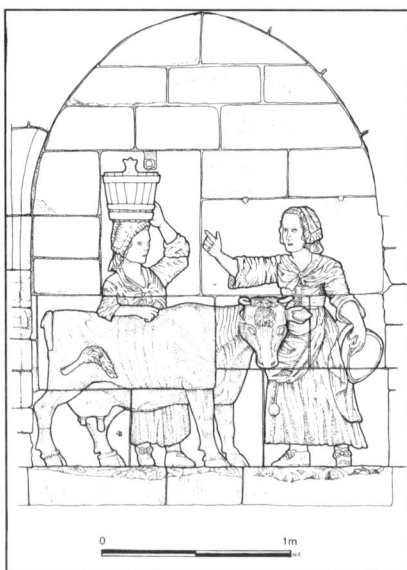

Figure 4.2. Dun Cow sculpture group on Durham Cathedral (Norman Emery, Cathedral Archaeologist).

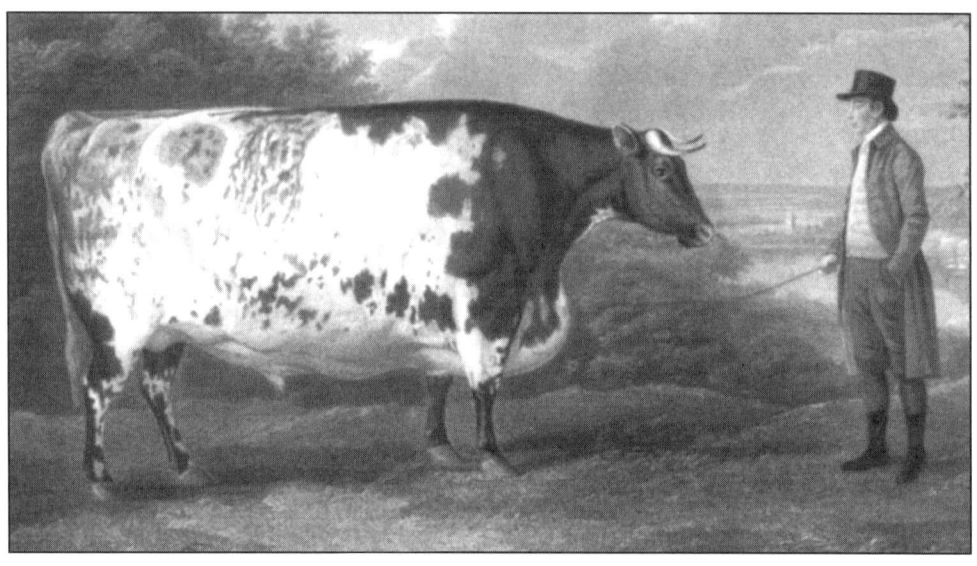

Figure 4.3. The Durham Ox: detail of painting by Boultbee.

requirement by the standards of the mid twentieth century (Morley 1950). The sculptor was clearly sympathetic to, and knowledgeable about, dairy cows, as the Dun Cow is so lifelike she could be a portrait of a real animal. The Dun Cow may be taken as an instantly recognizable image of a dairy cow in the later eighteenth century: small, lean and with an excellent udder.

So, the question arises of how long the small native cattle coexisted with the new improved cattle. Authors of the time, busy promoting the large cattle, were dismissive of the small ones. Bewick (1980, 28), for example, noted that 'our horned cattle are universally allowed to be the finest in Europe; although such as are purely British are inferior in size'.

There are some clues that explain the survival of these small cattle alongside the large ones. One is the presence of minor abnormalities (exostoses) on the distal (lower) ends of the bones of the small cattle from both Alnwick and Whitby, but not on the bones of the large ones. Similar changes have been seen on the same lower leg bones from draught oxen (Bartosiewicz *et al.* 1997). This does not mean that these small cattle were oxen, but rather that they probably did a lot of walking, possibly on rough ground, during their lifetime. Winchester (2000) has shown that, though in decline, traditional patterns of shieling, or sending the cows up to the hill pastures in the summer months, survived into the post-medieval period. It is possible that the small bones from Alnwick and Whitby, with hill pastures in the hinterland, represent the marketing of cull cows from such a system of husbandry. The large fat oxen would not have been immediately attractive to the hill farmers of the region, interested in producing butter and cheese from steep pastures and poor quality grazing.

The eighteenth century is well known as an age of agricultural improvement. Bakewell's ideas on livestock breeding were very influential, with both the Culley and Colling brothers studying his methods first hand and disseminating these practices in the north-east. For example, George Culley contributed largely to the *General View of the Agriculture of Northumberland, Cumberland and Westmoreland* (Bailey 1810). The Culley brothers farmed leased estates in Northumberland, besides the family property in Co. Durham, and regularly sent stock south to be fattened and sold from the Durham farm at Denton. Livestock from the Culleys' holdings were traded at markets as far afield as Berwick and Yorkshire (Orde 2004). The Colling brothers of Ketton Hall and Barmpton, near Darlington, were pre-eminent in breeding improved shorthorn cattle. Their stock realized phenomenal prices for the time, with buyers from all over the north of England. The Durham Ox was bred by the Collings but the lasting fame of this animal is due to John Day, who purchased the Ox and exhibited him throughout the country from 1801–1807 (Comben 2007). This remarkable progress, of over 3,000 miles, was unique propaganda for the improved Durham Shorthorns, and is commemorated along the route of his travels by public houses named after the Durham Ox, with an example at Beeston near Nottingham, close to the conference venue at which this paper was presented. In 1817, only ten years after the death of the Durham Ox, cattle of this improved type, explicitly bred on the river Tees, were exported to Kentucky (Henlein 1959, 29–30).

The sudden appearance, archaeologically, of these large post-medieval cattle is linked to a combination of factors. There was a rising demand for meat from an increasing and prosperous urban and industrial population, such as the colliers and seamen associated with the Tyne and Wear. The enclosures brought an end to traditional husbandry by placing control of decision-making over large acreages in the hands of a few prosperous and articulate people, allowing the introduction of new fodder crops and controlled breeding of livestock. The ox was being widely replaced by the horse as an agricultural draught animal (Langdon 1986). The Durham Ox, for instance, would not have been as fat had he been worked in the yoke.

The type of small, lean dairy cow, as exemplified by the Dun Cow, was unsuited to meet the new market for beef. The progressive farmers of the region therefore responded to this consumer-led demand by the creation of large animals, to improve carcase size, meat yield and profit. Some of this increase in size may be attributed to changes in breeding policy. One of the most famous Shorthorn bulls, Comet, bred by Charles Colling, was closely in-bred. Imported livestock also contributed to the genetics of these large animals. Bailey (1810, 226) particularly mentions a Mr Michael Dobinson of Sedgefield, 'who brought a bull out of Holland that is said to have improved the breed'. Continental Europe has a tradition of breeds larger than those native to Britain.

The people breeding these large cattle in the late eighteenth century were prosperous men, who could afford to experiment with new ideas of cultivation and stock raising. It is also salutary to note that some, such as Robert Colling and Charles Forster, were single gentlemen. These men were what would now be termed 'agribusinessmen', intentionally producing large quantities of meat as a commodity product for an urban market and delegating the hands-on management of their farms to stewards. It is very clear that they had no interest in, or use for, cows for the dairy or the women needed to run a dairy. For example, Orde (2004, 332) notes that the Culleys were not dairy farmers, were unfamiliar with the market for butter or dealing in it and so lost money when selling surplus butter from their house cows. This would have been unthinkable two centuries earlier to educated gentleman farmers and agricultural writers like Thomas Tusser and Gervaise Markham, who expected their wives and daughters to have hands on practical experience in the dairy, amongst other skills.

Cobbett (2001, 330), writing in 1830, was of the opinion that 'a fat ox is a finer thing than a cheese, however good.' This attitude appears to have been endemic at the time and crossed with the settlers to the cattle-ranching states of America, who were:

> indifferent toward dairying. The production of dairy items required too much skilled labour, it was thought, and hence would not pay. Many of the cattlemen could not possibly envision themselves tending 'milch cows', traditionally the task of the farmwife and children. (Henlein 1959, 68–9)

The Dun Cow and the Durham Ox

Prior to the railways, there was no way of supplying an urban market for liquid milk from remote rural pastures. The manufacture of milk into butter and cheese was therefore essential. The high labour inputs for low financial returns from dairy cattle, like the Dun Cow, and the converse for fat beef cattle, like the Durham Ox, hastened the demise of the small cattle. The association of the Dun Cow with the dairymaids underlines the dichotomy between the new large beef animals, bred by articulate, wealthy men with multiple holdings, and the small dairy cows suited to small, family-run, farmsteads, where the women were still intimately involved in the decision-making concerning the cattle. The class and gender divide therefore worked against the interests of the small cattle that had been bred for untold generations to suit the local country. Though in decline, Bailey (1810, 236) noted that 'the variety of great milkers is yet to be found wherever the dairy is the chief object'. By 1859, Darwin (1994, 86) describes the ancient black cattle of Yorkshire as having been first supplanted by the Longhorns and then 'swept away by the short-horns (I quote the words of an agricultural writer) as if by some murderous pestilence'.

The success of the large fat cattle in the north-east was in part due to environmental determinism. The land was suited to growing the quantities of fodder needed to maintain fat oxen. Cobbett, on his northern tour in 1832, was amazed by the productivity of the grassland he saw, and graphically described the amount of fodder necessary to maintain a fat ox in southern England:

> we know that we might put an ox up to his eyes in our grass, and that it would only just keep him from growing worse: we know that we are obliged to have turnips and meal and cabbages and parsnips and potatoes, and then, with some of our hungry hay for them to pick their teeth with, we make shift to put fat upon an ox. (Cole and Cole 1930, 699)

It is known today that heavy cattle are by their nature inefficient feed converters and are only profitable when there is a demand for large joints (Long 2006).

Rogers (2004, 40–55) chronicles the increasing association during the eighteenth century between roast beef and patriotism in response to the political threat from France. The provisioning of the armed forces during the Napoleonic Wars created a further demand for large quantities of beef. It should be noted here that the finds of the large and small cattle bones from Whitby came from the infill of a dry dock constructed at this time. The subsequent post-war depression saw many farmers, who had followed the farming practices advocated by improvers like the Culleys and Collings, tied to long leases and high rents and facing bankruptcy. Fat oxen became hobby animals for the wealthy and the aristocracy, endorsed by the royal family. Prince Albert's entries at Smithfield show were regular prize winners. These monstrous animals were a continuing object of satire in Punch and their eating qualities roundly denounced by Meg Dods (1988, 93): 'Fashion and luxury have lately introduced stall-fed oxen, which are better fitted to the tallow-chandler than the cook. They are indeed good for nothing, save to obtain premiums at Cattle-shews, and deluge dripping-pans with liquid fat.' Meg Dods, however, was cook for the epicures of the Cleikum Club. The keel men and colliers of the Tyne, engaged in heavy manual labour, were probably more appreciative of the suet and dripping associated with fat beef.

The widespread disappearance of the small native dairy cow left a gap in the market when a demand arose in the mid-nineteenth century for small house cows for middle class families. Imported Breton cattle from France, and then Kerry and Dexter cattle from Ireland, filled this niche. The Dexter was the most successful of these imports, with Edward VII being president of the Dexter Cattle Society 1901–2. One does wonder whether his patronage of this diminutive breed was a reaction to the monstrous fat oxen bred by his father! Baker and Manwell (1987, 177) chronicle the rise and fall in popularity of the Breton cattle and 'the important roles played by fads, fashion, agribusiness pressures and breed society interests, all superimposed upon changing economic and social patterns', rather than any lack of biological or economic fitness on the part of the animals. Many of the same factors that led to the failure of the introduced Breton had previously contributed to the extermination of the small native cattle.

The Durham Shorthorn cattle were bred during the nineteenth century into several distinct types. The modern beef Shorthorn retains the stature of the large, early, improved animals. The Northern Dairy Shorthorn is now a rare breed but was the dairy cow of the Pennine Dales. It seems probable that the Northern Dairy Shorthorn incorporated, by cross breeding, the milking qualities of the small local cattle that had adapted to the pastures of Northumberland and Durham over many centuries.

Until the eighteenth century, the cattle bones found on archaeological sites do show some evidence of regional variation and differences in size but these are minor compared to the sudden, and previously unprecedented, appearance of the massive bones from improved later eighteenth-century cattle. The integration of these large animals into farming systems and the major change in the type and quality of beef produced are topics that are rarely considered by archaeologists. This paper has endeavoured to demonstrate the broader understanding of the change in diet that can be obtained by using sources of information from other disciplines.

References

Archaeological Services. 2006. *Alnwick Castle, Alnwick, Northumberland: Archaeological Monitoring.* (Unpublished report no. 1502, Archaeological Services Durham University).

Bailey, J. 1810. *General View of the Agriculture of Northumberland, Cumberland and Westmoreland* (London).

Baker, C.M.A. and Manwell C. 1987. 'The Breton breed of cattle in Britain: extinction versus fitness', *Agricultural History Review* **35**, 171–78.

Bartosiewicz, L., Van Neer, W. and Lentacker, A. 1997. *Draught Cattle: Their Osteological Identification and History* (Tervuren, Annales Sciences Zoologiques 281).

Bewick, T. 1980 facsimile of 1807. *A General History of Quadrupeds* (Leicester).

Cobbett, W. 2001 reprint of 1830. *Rural Rides* (Harmondsworth).

Cole, G.D.H. and Cole, M. 1930. *Cobbett's Rural Rides 3* (London).

Comben, N. 2007. *The Durham Ox* (Nottingham).

Darwin, C. 1994 facsimile of 1872. *The Origin of Species* (London).

Dods, M. 1988 facsimile of 1829. *The Cook and Housewife's Manual* (London).

Gidney, L.J. 2002. *Whitby UWWTD Scheme: Church Street. Animal Bone Assessment* (Unpublished Northern Archaeological Associates Report 2002/71).

Henlein, P.C. 1959. *Cattle Kingdom in the Ohio Valley 1783–1860* (Lexington).

Langdon, J. 1986. *Horses, Oxen and Technological Innovation* (Cambridge).

Long, J. 2006. 'Demand for larger joints sees finishing weight rise', *Farmers Weekly* 20/10/06, 42.

Morley, A. 1950. *Dairy Farmers Encyclopaedia* (Kingswood).

Orde, A. 2004. 'The Culleys and Farm Management', *Northern History* **41**, 327–338.

Rogers, B. 2004. *Beef and Liberty* (London).

Stallibrass, S. 1993. 'Post-Medieval cattle burials from St Giles by Brompton Bridge, North Yorkshire', *English Heritage Ancient Monuments Laboratory Report 94/93* (London).

Stokes, P.R.G. and Huntley, J.P. 1998. 'Animal bone from Market Place, Masham', *Durham Environmental Archaeology Report 57/98*.

Winchester, A.J.L. 2000. *The Harvest of the Hills* (Edinburgh).

'A Moveable Feast': Negotiating Gender at the Middle-Class Tea-Table in Eighteenth- and Nineteenth-Century England

Annie Gray,
University of Liverpool

A cup of tea…says to the brain, 'now rise, and show your strength. Be eloquent, and deep, and tender; see, with a clear eye, into Nature, and into life: spread your white wings of quivering thought and soar, a god-like spirit over the whirling world beneath you'. (Jerome 1994, 92–3)

The integration of tea into the English psyche is such that it has willingly been adapted as part of the national stereotype. Anglicized tea rituals and material culture are part of the culture anywhere the English have left their mark. Although the artefacts associated with tea – notably easily broken and equally easily identifiable ceramics – are often examined by archaeologists, tea itself has rarely been treated with the attention it deserves, either by archaeologists or food historians. It has a fascinating trajectory, from its beginnings as an elite, minority and frankly alien drink in the mid seventeenth century to lending its name to a meal eaten by the early twentieth-century working classes. Throughout much of its history tea has been closely identified with women, a link which continues to be made to this day by the less innovative elements of the advertising industry.

Archaeology and tea
Within archaeology ceramics in general and teawares in particular have overwhelmingly been used for quantitative analysis. The very ubiquity of teawares at historical sites has seen them become important sources for dating and, as such, they are often included in site analyses. However, while such data is important for analytical studies of areas and social groups, it is not without its pitfalls. Led by George Miller (1988; 1991), the study of ceramics has produced a number of monographs on pricing, theoretically of use in assigning social status. However, more recent work has suggested that such generalizations can be unhelpful, especially since goods could be acquired through a variety of ways including theft, loans, gifts and the purchase of seconds or thirds directly or indirectly from factories (Ewins 1997). Work based on pattern books has illustrated that consumer choice was wide and could be used to demonstrate (or negate) lifestyle choices and beliefs (Brooks 1999; Lucas 2003). Recognition of the polysemous nature of objects, including dining and teawares, has led to more qualitatively analytical studies,

demonstrating that choice of pattern and style involved more than just economics, and that ceramics may be the key to investigating class and gender (DiZerega Wall 1994). Yet while some of these studies include teawares there has been no in-depth theoretically-informed examination of the development of tea-taking in either America or the UK. Ceramics and other material culture linked to tea are usually considered alongside dining ephemera (e.g. Brooks 1999; Lucas 2003) and when considered separately they are assigned meanings based on class, discipline and emulation (Brighton 2001; Shackel 1993). One exception to this is DiZerega Wall's (1994) *Archaeology of Gender*, which places teawares and other ceramic goods in an engendered context and uses them to explore changes within the urban middle class household in America in the early nineteenth century. This paper seeks to address issues raised by the use of teawares in an English context without awareness of the historical development of tea-drinking, problematizing the assumed association between women and tea ceremony and adding nuances to what seems at first to be a straightforward emulative model.

Teawares were associated with and predominantly bought by women as consumers in their own right (DiZerega Wall 1994, 135). Studies of consumer lists indicate large one-off ceramic sales were often to men, while sales of everyday and cheaper items were arranged by women (Vickery and Styles 2006, 26). Equally, historical consideration of diaries, estate books and letters indicate that by at least the mid eighteenth century women controlled tea-related purchases (Vickery 1998), just as they had taken control of the tea ceremony itself. An understanding of the dynamics of tea-drinking therefore has significant implications for considering gender relations in the context both of the household and the wider world.

The period from the introduction of tea in England (*c.*1650) to 1900 can roughly be divided into three phases: *c.*1650–1750 during which tea was a minority drink considered by some to carry significant health risks; *c.*1750–1830 when tea gained great popularity, dropped in price and became a drink for all despite disapproval from the elites; and *c.*1830–1900 by when tea was regarded as fuel for living, displacing beer as the drink of the masses (Burnett 1966). At first glance this is a classic journey from luxury to necessity but, as will be seen, though tea drinking itself follows this model, its associated material culture and meanings differed depending on social and gender context.

During the first phase of the introduction of tea, it was viewed as an adjunct to the far more popular coffee and indeed chocolate, and was served like them at the male-dominated coffee houses. As with coffee and chocolate, tea was the subject of often vitriolic treatises prophesying impotence, still births and similar misfortune to those who partook (Duncan 1706). Despite this, by the 1750s it had become established as part of the upper class English diet. It had also developed not only an instantly recognizable set of material culture associated with the English way of taking tea and owing very little to its Chinese origins, but also an associated time-slot – the mid-afternoon (though this was by no means the only time tea was consumed). Both of these characteristics came together in the form of the English tea ceremony, with the usual set of indefinable and rapidly-changing rules which served to confuse foreigners, much to the delight of contemporary satirists. Meanwhile tea also got cheaper, or at least bastardized forms of it did (Anon. 1978, 281). By the 1784 Commutation Act the government had recognized that, '*tea has become an economical substitute to the Middle and Lower Classes for malt liquor, the price of which renders it impossible to procure the quantity sufficient for them as their only drink*' (Emmerson 1992, 11).

During the nineteenth century tea grew in popularity to the extent that the British Government deemed it an investment opportunity and cultivated tea plantations in its territories in India. Profits and quantity quickly eclipsed Chinese imports (Pettigrew 2001, 89) and tea remains synonymous with India to this day. The afternoon tea ceremony lost its aristocratic associations although remaining a significant occasion for predominantly female sociability in leisured society. Afternoon Tea as 'invented' by the Victorians – the inevitable creation myth hinges on the Duchess of Bedford's moment of hunger in 1841 – was a continuum of an established custom going back to the eighteenth century, given a new name by cookbook writers seeking to give it a more approachable form. Other occasions for drinking tea were of course still present, and Beeton's mammoth edition of *c.*1888 lists five different types of tea-as-meal including 'old-fashioned' and 'quiet' teas (Beeton 1888, 1439). Class played a huge role in determining the name of one's tea-based meal, and arguably still does today.

Love and scandal: 1700–1750

The painting by van Aken illustrated overleaf is typical of early depictions of the English at tea. The presence of the beverage is an indication of the wealth and taste of the family. It is also indicative of links to the wider – imperial – world. At this early stage tea and Englishness were not yet synonymous, and the display of tea shows pride in late Stuart and Georgian empire building as well as an assumption that this will continue (Lawson 1997). The equipage of tea is shown in loving detail – the lockable tea caddy kept securely by the mistress' feet, the silverware on the table and the redware teapot – either Chinese or by the Dutch Elers brothers working in Vauxhall. Tea is not the only drink present; the servant on the right carries a chocolate pot and the elongated shape of the cups which echo the early cocoa pod cups also indicates chocolate consumption.

The domestic setting is characteristic of depictions of tea in this era. Despite consumption in public and semi-public spaces such as coffee houses and booths, tea rapidly became associated with the home and through that with women. Reasons are partly linked to the growth of the tea equipage itself and it is difficult to untangle the rise in availability of ceramic tea goods from the increasing association of tea with a context in which such items could be used with less fear of breakage than that of the coffee house. China was already associated with women by the 1670s (Kowaleski-Wallace 1995, 52–57), and the development of ceramic tea assemblages extended that link to tea. Tea had advantages over coffee and chocolate in a domestic setting, including the

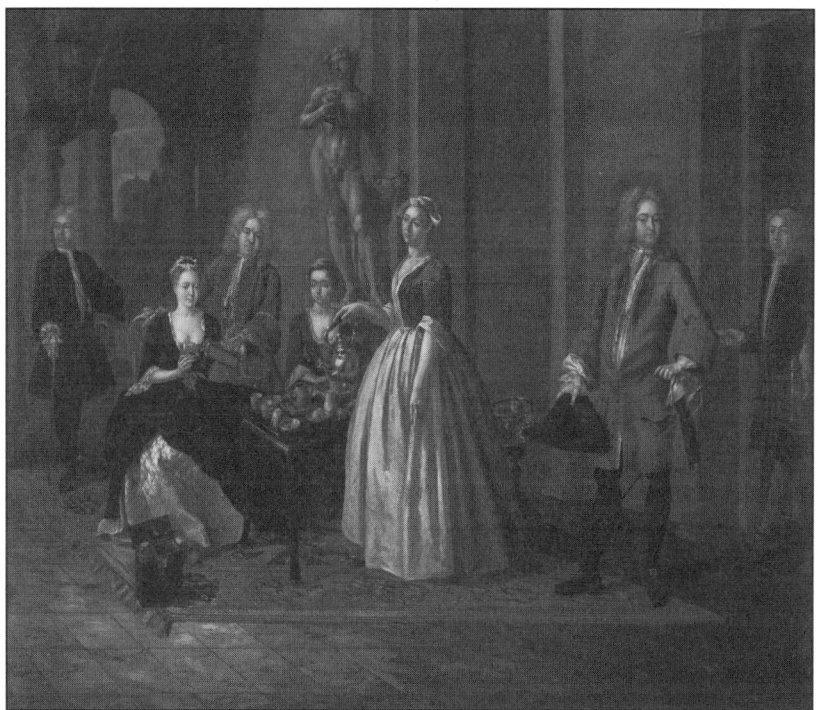

Figure 5.1. J. van Aken, An English Family at Tea *(c.1720). (Photograph © Tate Britain)*

psychological one of control. Tea leaves, unlike cocoa or coffee beans, did not need to be taken to the kitchen to be processed. They could be kept under lock and key and in the possession of the mistress and through this used, as in Figure 5.1, to demonstrate status. Both coffee and chocolate were also expensive, and yet rarely associated with lockable caddies. Tea on the other hand made the holder of the key – the mistress – the focal point at gatherings where tea was consumed. This was a significant way in which to gain influence and notice in the domestic context and a reason for feminine privileging of tea in the home.

Women therefore had a vested interest in promoting tea drinking. The late seventeenth century was a period where women had a rare glimpse of a less misogynistic world, and in which a few female writers were able to be taken seriously, touting the beginnings of what would later be termed feminist ideas (Clery 2004). Arguments over perceptions and the role of women in the period have been well-rehearsed elsewhere so this paper will assume at least a passing familiarity with them.

Despite the recognition of – limited – female worth, not everyone was supportive of the concept of women presiding over tea-parties and forging a significant role in the social landscape of the home. This landscape, it should be remembered, was just as important as any coffee house, both in terms of female social and business networks and also as a site for family-based networking. The link between women and china previously mentioned was largely a negative one (e.g. Wycherley 2001). China was often used as a metaphor for virtue, and Hogarth especially used broken vases at the feet of seemingly elegant young women to denote that more than just the vase was no longer intact. China broke easily – one reason it was prized was that the correct handling of it could be used to show familiarity and therefore wealth and class. But it could also be seen as an expensive waste versus clothing or housing improvements (Richards 1999). When tea was added as a third element the satirists took great glee in using the tea-table as a metaphor for wasted time and the encouragement of idleness. Worse still, by involving men in their tea-taking, women could be accused of active engagement in the corruption of the virtuous world. Such ideas took hold rapidly. Already in 1694 Congreve felt able to refer to women retiring to their '*tea and scandal, according to their ancient custom*' (Congreve 1996).

The developing equipage

The tea equipage is familiar to anyone working in this period, or indeed anyone with familiarity with art history museums such as the V&A. However, although there is a tendency to take the range of equipment for granted there is no intrinsic reason why, of the three hot beverages introduced in the seventeenth century, tea alone should so quickly and enduringly have gained an associated and distinctive set of material culture. The basic needs of all three beverages are the same – a container to hold the raw material, a vessel in which to make it and a cup from which to drink it. Dufour (1681) notes very little else in his description of how to make tea. Yet by 1750 the material culture of tea encompassed cups, saucers, up to three different types of spoons, sugar tongs, sugar boxes and bowls, milk and hot water jugs, caddies, slop bowls, plates for any edible accompaniments and of course the teapot itself (Pettigrew 2003). One reason for this, as explained above, is the association with a domestic setting. Once tea-taking became frequent away from robust public spaces the increasingly ceramic-based equipage could safely expand, driven by entrepreneurs seeing opportunities for sales and the purchasers who happily believed that slop bowls were indispensible.

Tea by the 1750s had become an instrument of female sociability, and it has been argued that teas took the place of the coffee house in female circles (Clery 1991). Far more useful than trying to locate specifically female forms of sociability, however, is to view tea-taking as a gendered addition to the corpus of occasions on which social networks could be maintained by both men and women. Tea was a feminized, domestic occasion. Both sexes partook of tea, but it was women who wielded the teapot. The proliferation of specialist equipment was therefore one way in which to combat negative views of women as a whole. Far from encouraging chit-chat, indolence and immorality, women were able to use their familiarity with a range of delicate objects as a means of enforcing genteel behaviours and of representing their unbroken virtue. Slowly a discourse emerged in which women were a disciplining force over uncouth man, presiding over a domestic sociability in which habits of hard work and good manners could be encouraged (Clery 2004).

Tea and sociability: c.1750–1830

By 1750, tea was accepted as part of the English diet. It was in this period that tea started to become part of the English national stereotype. By the end of it tea as a cooking ingredient had virtually disappeared from cookbooks as the increasing segmentation of material things saw it labelled as 'drink' rather than 'food'. Tea was no longer included as an indicator of wealth and taste in portraiture as its consumption, albeit often heavily adulterated, descended down the social scale. Satirists played on fears of emulation, while social reformers alternatively lauded it as an alternative to gin or denounced it as a waste of a meagre budget (Emmerson 1992). Suggestions as to why it attained such overwhelming popularity range from the actions of the East India Company (Chaudhuri 1978) through market forces to the use of tea as a means of consuming sugar (Brown 1995, 56; Mintz 1985). It is probable that many factors influenced take-up of tea, not the least of which was its versatility.

Tea was drunk on a number of occasions, including in the afternoons, after meals, at tea gardens and as part of the round of garden-admiring of large house-parties. Women continued to play an integral role and diaries such as those of the Rev. Penrose (Penrose *et al.* 1983) clearly indicate that the female-led opportunity to take tea with acquaintances was key to sociability. The Victorian notion of a woman, at least for the middle classes, was domestic, gentle and able to act as a guiding force for her family and husband. While the notion of a strict public/private divide has long since been discredited, gender roles were nevertheless prescribed and ideals set up which assimilated the idea of women as able to control her immediate environment just as she had demonstrated control over the tea table.

There was a huge choice of tea equipage by the early nineteenth century. The ideal set as seen in early seventeenth-century paintings remained unchanged, though by the 1820s teabowls were more usually handled and called cups. By the nineteenth century matching sets can be seen in makers' catalogues although it is more usual to find the

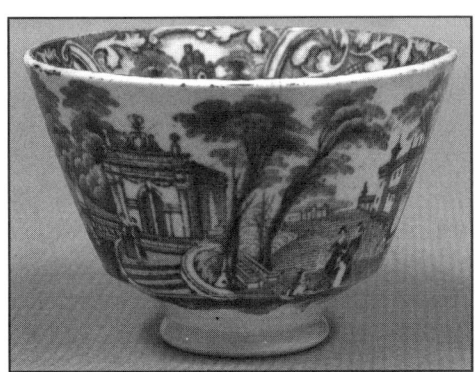

Figure 5.2. Teabowl, c.1820s. Cheap transfer-printed scene showing figures in contemporary dress promenading through a wooded landscape, complete with classical ruins. Unknown maker. (Photo by author, reproduced courtesy of York Museums Trust [YORCH: 161.74])

various elements sold separately (e.g. Don Pottery 1983) and it is likely that the majority of consumers had small sets which they put together as the occasion arose. The teapot was a focal point; by its nature it was better for displaying pattern and through that a measure of the mentality behind its choice. As English manufacturers geared up to cater for the market in teawares, modern marketing techniques became visible – the most notorious example being Wedgwood (Ewins 1997; McKendrick 1982). Choice of pattern included classical, bucolic, patriotic and oriental and could also include pointed political motifs as well as more personal touches. The buoyant market encouraged technological innovation and experimentation, with the result that early soft paste porcelain was rapidly eclipsed by bone china, and hand painted vessels increasingly lost market share to cheap transfer-printing (Figure 5.2).

While it is generally accepted that the most popular patterns in ceramic design were variations on the 'Chinese blue' at the turn of the eighteenth/nineteenth century (Lucas 2003, 129), it is possible to consider teapot designs in terms of the various elements which are present on pots. This can only be done using intact examples, either from pattern books or surviving examples in collections. Both of these sources have drawbacks as well as advantages, no more or less than archaeologically-recoverable data. Collection data enables the study of design as well as size and shape across a long period of time and demonstrates the sheer variety of designs on offer. Taking the latter as a data set and assigning up to three design categories to each pot, analysis suggests that the most commonly found motif on teapots between 1780 and 1820 was floral. Flowers were often incorporated into landscape or domestic scene-based designs, for example as a border or single element featuring on the spout, lid or handle. In a data set of 308 teapots dating to 1750–1900 at least 50 per cent contained floral elements in any one decade, rising to 78 per cent and 82 per cent for the periods 1800–1809 and 1810–1819 respectively. The majority of these were polychrome designs. Whether this indicates that blue monochrome is over-represented in excavated data or under-represented in museum collections is uncertain.

This may be deemed an 'obvious' feminine pattern, fitting with the popularity of floral fabrics and designs in ladies magazines. Yet while floral and faunal elements are less overtly politicized than other possible choices, and may represent a retreat from the wars and domestic turmoil of the period, they also reflect one of the tensions in nineteenth-century society: between domesticated and wild. Beeton's (2000, 363–372) tremulous yet excited descriptions of the hog are just one example from another sphere (Buzard 1997). Floral designs represent the taming of nature and the bringing under control of a tumultuous society. Floral elements within other designs carried the same meaning. As peace returned to Britain in the 1820s other designs once more become popular (although floral motifs continue to be the single most common element in teapot design).

'A Moveable Feast'

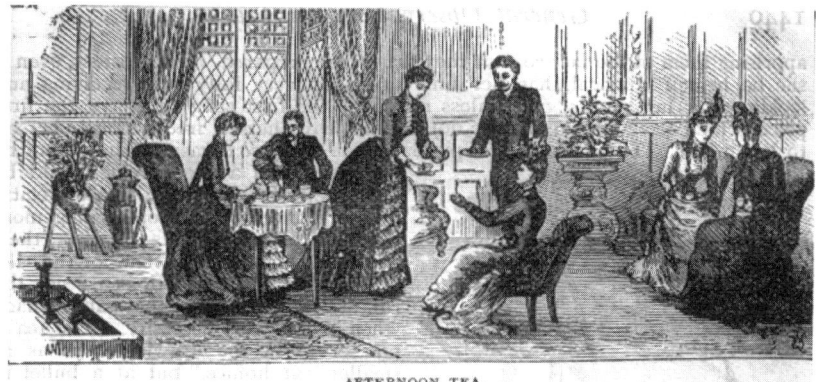

Figure 5.3. Middle-class afternoon tea. The archaeologically familiar paraphernalia of domesticity abounds – flowerpots, knick-knacks, and the tea service itself. (Beeton 1888, 1439)

A universal drink: c.1830–1900

As the nineteenth century progressed it is remarkable how ubiquitous tea became. It was drunk at every social level, and each class had its own specific tea consumption occasions – in addition, that is, to the chain-drinking of tea which was as familiar a habit then as now. For the upper classes the tea ceremony became fixed around mid-afternoon, an ideal time for informal entertaining, enabling staff to prepare small dishes and clear the rooms involved before the preparation for dinner began. From the 1870s references start to occur in number to afternoon tea. This was driven by the vast quantity of guidance books struggling for differentiation in a crowded marketplace and the codification of food and dining as previously unexplored eating and drinking occasions were set down in print. The middle classes embraced afternoon tea and depictions of tea on the lawn or in the drawing room bear a striking resemblance to the conversation pieces of 200 years before.

Commemoration teas were a further example of tea-as-national-emblem as well as enabling the middle-class organizers to impose their view of a correctly ordered society on the lower classes. Essentially showcases for male egos, thinly disguised as philanthropic gestures, they relied on women to wield the teapot and with it dish out helpings of middle-class work ethics. Accounts of their planning indicate the bickering and self-interest that underlay the events, as well as demonstrating the assigning of roles according to gender: men formed the committees, procured ingredients, supervised cooking and tasted the beer; women wore flowers and poured the tea (Anon. 1887a; 1887b). Control was paramount, and invitees divided along lines of age and parish. In the case of Cambridge's coronation feast, tables were laid out in a spiral from a raised central platform: an arrangement not unlike the panopticon structures favoured by institutional building designers (Hallack 1838). In this context, the role of women as a controlling force within the domestic environment was accepted and promoted through the medium of tea.

'A Moveable Feast'

In the eighteenth century women appropriated the material culture of tea to fight for a responsible role in society – a role which they won. By the end of the nineteenth century the view of the ideal middle class women as mother, wife and role model had itself become limiting. Women could be perceived as passive and inward-looking, and the growing market in souvenir teawares further cast women as a repository of memories, a role still automatically allotted to them – and accepted by them – by anthropologists in the twentieth century (Webster 1999). The relationship of femininity and tea by now was so strong that by the 1850s tea was used, predominantly by female authors, to explore traits and feelings not openly expressed in the text or understood by the characters. Subverting the comfortable domestic associations of tea, these ranged from women and witchcraft (Braddon 1986, 222) to sexual desire:

> She stood by the tea-table in a light-coloured muslin gown, which had a good deal of pink about it. She looked as if she was not attending to the conversation, but solely busy with the tea-cups, among which her round ivory hands moved with pretty, noiseless daintiness. She had a bracelet on one taper arm, which would fall down over her round wrist. Mr Thornton watched the re-placing of this troublesome ornament with far more attention than he listened to her father. *It seemed is if it fascinated him to see her push it up impatiently, until it tightened her soft flesh;* and then to mark the loosening – the fall. He could almost have exclaimed – 'There it goes again!' (Gaskell 1970, 120) [My italics]

It was also used as a tool by women in the gradual movement out of the home. Tearooms in towns, stations and on public transport mimicked the safe environment of the home, extending domesticity into public spaces and alleviating worries over travel and the dangers it could represent. Molly Hughes' (1946) accounts of her travels as a young teacher in the 1880s are peppered with references to tea on the move, creating a secure structure in which her unchaperoned self could move without fear of raising social indignation. Meanwhile the rise of town-centre tearooms from the 1890s (Pettigrew 2001, 134) afforded women a gendered space in which to socialize. For the middle classes this enabled women to end their suburban isolation and spend leisure time in areas which were by now predominantly places of work, not habitation (DiZerega Wall 1994). Increasingly tea provided a means of breaking down barriers as both middle and working class women became a more visible presence on the street now that they had a socially established and acceptable place to meet and socialize. This sociability has in turn been viewed as critical to the rise of women's suffrage and twentieth-century feminism (Pettigrew 2001, 136). Tea became a metaphor for home and stability, sustaining the illusion of the contented domesticated women while at the same time enabling women such as the early university students to survive the experiences that both shaped modern gender conventions and laid the groundwork for the opportunities we have today.

Acknowledgements

This study is funded by the AHRC. My thanks also to an anonymous referee who commented on an earlier draft of this paper.

References

Anonymous 1887a. *The Jubilee Celebrations of HM the Queen in Cambridge and Surrounding Villages, 1887*, Cambridge County Records Office.
Anonymous 1887b. *Wentworth Jubilee Celebrations, 1887*, Cambridge County Records Office.
Anonymous 1978. *Enquire Within Upon Everything* (London).
Beeton, I. 1888. *Mrs Beeton's Household Management* (London).
Beeton, I. 2000 facsimile of 1st edition of 1861. *The Book of Household Management* (London).
Braddon, M. 1986. *Lady Audley's Secret* (Oxford World's Classics).
Brighton, S. 2001. 'Prices that suit the times: shopping for ceramics at the Five Points', *Historical Archaeology* 35 (3), 16–30.
Brooks, A. 1999. 'Building Jerusalem: transfer printed finewares and the creation of British identity', in Tarlow, S. and West S. (ed.) *The Familiar Past? Archaeologies of Later Historical Britain* (London), 51–65.
Brown, P. 1995. *In Praise of Hot Liquors: The Study of Chocolate, Coffee and Tea-Drinking 1600–1850* (York).
Burnett, J. 1966. *Plenty and Want: A Social History of Diet in England from 1815 to the Present Day* (London).
Buzard, J. 1997. 'Home ec. with Mrs Beeton', *Raritan* 17 (2), 121–35.
Chaudhuri, K. 1978. *The Trading World of Asia and the English East India Company, 1660–1760* (Cambridge).
Clery, E. 1991. 'Women, publicity and the coffee house myth', *Women: A Cultural Review* 2 (2), 168–77.
Clery, E. 2004. *The Feminisation Debate in Eighteenth Century England: Literature, Commerce and Luxury* (Basingstoke).
Congreve, W. 1996. 'The Double-Dealer (1694)', in Partington, A. (ed.) *The Oxford Dictionary of Quotations* (Oxford), 214.
DiZerega Wall, D. 1994. *The Archaeology of Gender: Separating the Spheres in Urban America* (New York).
Don Pottery. 1983. *Pattern Book 1807* (Doncaster).
Dufour, P. 1681. *Traitez Nouveaux et Curieux du Café, du Thé et du Chocolat* (La Haye).
Duncan, Dr. 1706. *Wholesome Advice Against the Abuse of Hot Liquors* (London).
Emmerson, R. 1992. *British Teapots and Tea Drinking, 1700–1850* (London).
Ewins, N. 1997. '"Supplying the Present Wants of our Yankee Cousins…" Staffordshire Ceramics and the American Market, 1775–1880', *Journal of Ceramic History*, 15, 1–154.
Gaskell, E. 1970. *North and South* (Harmondsworth).
Hallack, T. 1838. *Origin and Progress and the Proceedings which ultimately led to the Coronation Dinner on Parker's Piece, Cambridge, June the 28th, 1838, on which occasion upwards of fifteen thousand persons dined together.* (Cambridge). This copy part of a bound volume including various other accounts of the same event and entitled 'Cambridge Coronation Festival 1838' (Cambridge University Library copy).
Hughes, M. 1946. *A London Family, 1870–1900*, 3 vols. (Oxford).
Jerome, J.K. 1994. *Three Men in a Boat* (London).
Kowaleski-Wallace, E. 1995. 'Women, china and consumer culture in eighteenth century England', *Eighteenth Century Studies* 29 (2), 153–67.
Lawson, P. 1997. 'Women and the empire of tea: image and counter-image in Hanoverian England', in Lawson, P. (ed.) *A Taste for Empire and Glory: Studies in British Overseas Expansion, 1660–1800* (Aldershot), chapter 15.
Lucas, G. 2003. 'Reading pottery: literature and transfer-printed pottery in the early nineteenth century', *International Journal of Historical Archaeology* 7 (2), 127–43.

McKendrick, N. 1982. 'Josiah Wedgwood and the commercialisation of the potteries', in McKendrick, N., J. Brewer and Plumb, J. (eds) *The Birth of a Consumer Society: The Commercialisation of Eighteenth Century England* (Bloomington), 100–145.

Miller, G. 1988: 'Classification and economic scaling of nineteenth century ceramics', in Beaudry, M. (ed.) *Documentary Archaeology in the New World* (Cambridge), 172–83.

Miller, G. 1991. 'A revised set of CC index values for classification and economic scaling of English ceramics from 1787–1880', *Historical Archaeology* **25** (1), 1–25.

Mintz, S. 1985. *Sweetness and Power: The Place of Sugar in Modern History* (New York).

Penrose, J., Mitchell, B. and Penrose, H. 1983. *Letters from Bath, 1766–1767 by the Rev. John Penrose* (Stroud).

Pettigrew, J. 2001. *A Social History of Tea* (London).

Pettigrew, J. 2003. *Design For Tea: Tea Wares from the Dragon Court to Afternoon Tea* (Stroud).

Richards, S. 1999. *Eighteenth Century Ceramics: Products for a Civilised Society* (Manchester).

Shackel, P. 1993. *Personal Discipline and Material Culture: An Archaeology of Annapolis, Maryland, 1695–1870* (Knoxville).

Vickery, A. 1998. *The Gentleman's Daughter: Women's Lives in Georgian England* (New Haven).

Vickery, A. and Styles, J. 2006. *Gender, Taste and Material Culture in Britain and North America, 1700–1830* (New Haven).

Webster, J. 1999. 'Resisting traditions: ceramics, identity and consumer choice in the Outer Hebrides from 1800 to the present', *International Journal of Historical Archaeology* **3** (1), 57–73.

Wycherley, W. 2001. *The Country Wife* (London).

The Economic, Social and Environmental Implications of Faunal Remains from the Bronze Age copper mines at Great Orme, North Wales

Sian James,
University of Liverpool

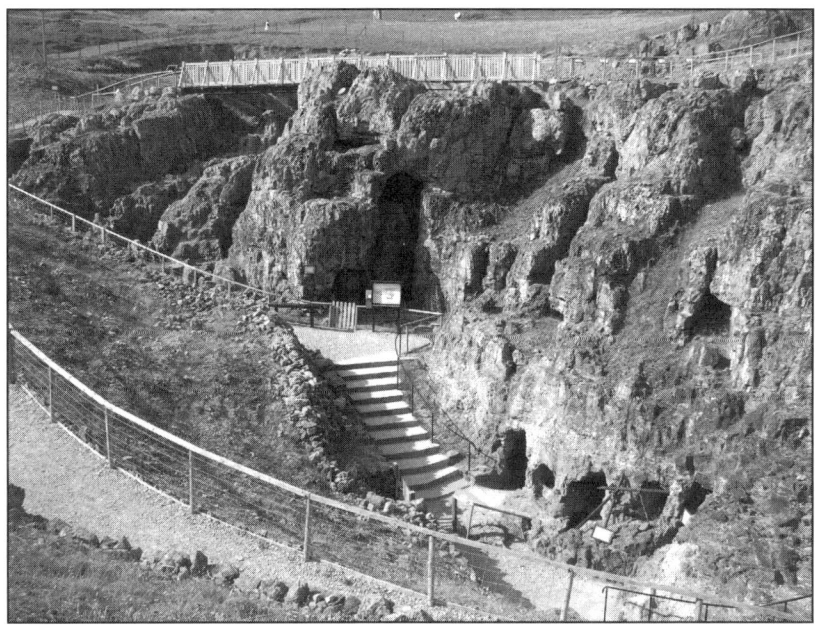

Figure 6.1. General view of the Great Orme Copper Mine, Llandudno (taken by the author).

Bronze Age European society is renowned for its metallurgy; however, the mechanisms by which metal ores were obtained, and in particular the lives of the people extracting them, have received little attention (Barber 2003, 79) compared to the more visible achievements of the period, for example monuments like Stonehenge, or indeed the metal artefacts themselves (Wager 2002, 105–6). The common criticism of archaeologists, when examining metalworking and mine sites, is that they appear to work in a 'contextual vacuum' (Pryor 2003, 273), looking at the artefacts and waste materials rather than the society and wider context. This paper will address this issue and shine a light on the underground activities on which Bronze Age society was built, by examining evidence for the diet and working practices of the individuals who created the Great Orme copper mines in Llandudno, North Wales. This is one of the largest prehistoric copper mining areas in the world: in the Pyllau Valley miles of tunnels have been uncovered revealing the wide-scale mining for copper ore that occurred from around 1900 BC (Figure 6.1). Recent excavations have yielded a unique and large collection of animal remains which has the potential to reveal how the miners were fed, as well as how food remains were themselves converted into mining tools. Here the evidence from Great Orme's faunal remains will be compared with data from other contemporary sites to theorize about the economic, social and environmental aspects surrounding the Bronze Age copper mines.

Background

The Great Orme is a peninsular of carboniferous limestone – 207 metres high, three kilometres long and over one and a half kilometres wide (Gravett and Jowett 1997, 1) – that overlooks the town of Llandudno in North Wales. The limestone was formed around 320 million years ago and subsequently fissures in the rock allowed copper-bearing minerals to seep through from deep within the earth's crust. The Great Orme mines have a long history of occupation evidenced by the archaeological and historical records. The greatest density of activity relates to the Bronze Age, which is the focus of this paper. Radiocarbon dates suggest that the mine was first opened around 1900 BC and was operational until about 1000 BC when the workers exhausted all the accessible ore, the remainder being below the water table where it stayed until being retrieved with the new mining technologies of the early eighteenth century (Lewis 1996, 35). In the late nineteenth century the mine was infilled and abandoned. It was only in the late 1980s that a survey by Ashton Mining Consultants led to the re-discovery of the Bronze Age network of tunnels and chambers (Lewis 1996, 43). Since then over five miles of tunnels have been discovered yielding two human bones, a few charcoal deposits, around 3000 stone hammers and, most significantly for this study, over 30,000 faunal remains. The mine is now run by Great Orme Mines Ltd who manage the site as a tourist attraction.

Evidence from animal bones

Most copper mines are acidic so the survival of animal remains is rare. Antler has been found at other mines throughout Europe, such as Cwmystwyth in Mid Wales (Timberlake 2003, 84), but this is often the only faunal evidence that survives. The zooarchaeological material from Great Orme is, admittedly, very fragmented due to both trampling and deliberate breakage but the mine's alkaline bedrock has enabled the survival of an exceptionally large assemblage. Several micro-studies have been carried out on aspects of the material (e.g. Hamilton-Dyer 1990, Wager 2002, 267) but, as part of my doctoral research, I have recorded and analysed over 16,000 animal bone fragments to date. These derive from mostly underground Bronze Age contexts, providing an excellent opportunity to study the role of animals in this sphere of prehistoric life.

In terms of species representation, cattle or cattle-sized animals comprise over 50 per cent of the assemblage, with sheep/goat and pig making up most of the remainder. Many of these domesticate bones exhibit butchery marks indicative of disarticulation, with some possible evidence for marrow extraction. It would seem that, as suggested by Hamilton-Dyer (1990, 4), most of the remains represent food waste. However, the assemblage also contains a few dog and horse bones – none of these demonstrated butchery marks and so it is debatable whether their flesh was consumed by people. Both red and roe deer post-cranial bones are represented in low frequencies, suggesting that wild mammals were occasionally hunted. There is no indication that wildfowl or fish were exploited, their bones being absent from the assemblage. A few mussel shells and one oyster shell are present, indicating that the nearby coastal resources were utilized to some extent (certainly the large number of granite stone cobbles must have been brought from the beach). It is possible that the dearth of bird and fish remains is due to recovery bias; however, I have carried out sieving experiments on newly-excavated deposits and the absence of these vertebrate categories appears to be genuine.

Skeletal patterning for the mammal remains demonstrates an over-representation of meat-bearing elements, in particular long bones and ribs (Figure 6.2). There is a distinct lack of skull and foot bones (metapodia), suggesting that primary butchery, which would have removed these 'low-utility' elements, happened away from the mine. Very few articulated remains have been discovered, although a sheep skeleton was found amongst the Bronze Age deposits (Lewis 1996, Appendix C7). With this one exception, the data suggest that, unsurprisingly, the miners transported the animal remains as small, pre-butchered portions rather than as complete carcasses.

Mining is a strenuous occupation that traditionally requires a high calorific diet to enable workers to toil long hours in cramped conditions (Wager 2002, 88). It may be assumed that many of the bones recovered from Great Orme represent the Bronze Age equivalents of pasties (such as those popularized by Cornish tin-miners), with miners taking cuts of meat to sustain them during their 'shift' in the cold, damp mine; the meat being consumed and the bones discarded. Demand for calories may also explain why some of the bones had been smashed, the workers perhaps trying to gain access to the marrow: Outram (2002, 51) has shown this to be an important source of fat, particularly valued by hunter-gatherer societies.

An alternative explanation for the high percentage of fragmented bones could be that they were ritually broken within the mine, perhaps used as closing or termination deposits for certain tunnels. Bone implements may have been left as offerings comparable to the historical miners' belief in 'knockers' or old miners who would cause mischief underground if not appeased by gifts (Lewis 1996, 129). The contemporary site of Grimes Graves in Norfolk has flint mine shafts covered with complete and broken antler tools before it was abandoned (Clutton-Brock 1984, 9). The rationale for such underground rituals is difficult to discern and has been the subject of many studies (Bradley 2000; Beecroft 2005), but it seems plausible that Bronze Age miners felt that, if they were taking something from the earth, they ought to give something in return. It may be for this reason that the sheep skeleton was deposited – sheep often being used for sacrifice in the past (Palmer 2001, 274). A ritual interpretation may also be proffered for the stone cobbles found at the end of tunnels; similar examples have been discovered in Continental European Bronze Age mines such as Rudna Glava, Serbia (Jovanović 1980, 34).

Prior to their deposition, the quartz cobbles were probably used as stone hammers for pounding the softer limestone. Certainly many of the animal bones were put to use as mining tools: of the 2489 bones that Hamilton-Dyer and Hunt analysed, 91 (3 per cent) were recognized as tools (Wager 2002, 267). My study reveals that 5 per cent of bones are probable tools, rising to 10 per cent if possible tools are included. These include long bones and ribs demonstrating rounded ends (Figure 6.2), worn from picking out the copper ore, whereas shoulder blades exhibit wear patterns consistent with having been used as shovels. I have replicated these various use–wear patterns during experiments using cattle and sheep bones as tools in the mine.

Great Orme in context

The significance of the Great Orme faunal assemblage can only be gauged by comparison with animal bone deposits from other contemporary sites, both industrial (e.g. other mines) and domestic, in the region. Unfortunately, there are few similarly-dated settlement sites in close proximity to the Great Orme mine, the only examples being an ore processing site Ffynnon Galchog (Lewis 1996), and a small smelting site (Website 1).

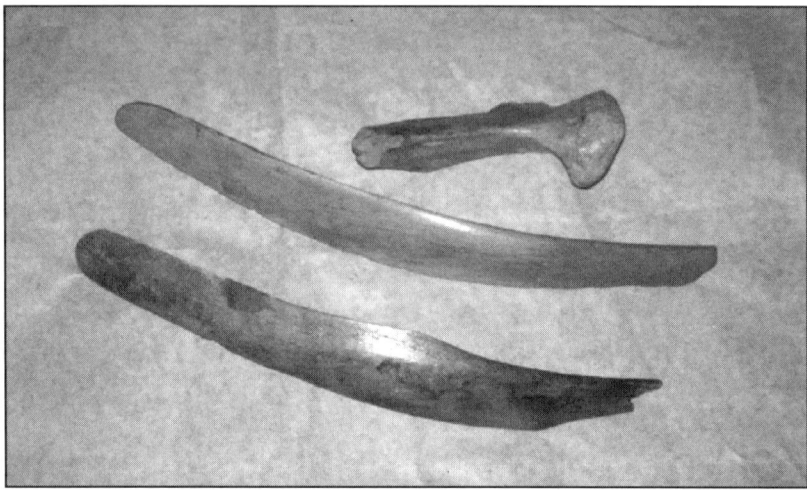

Figure 6.2. Bone tools from Great Orme copper mine (photo by H. Jowett).

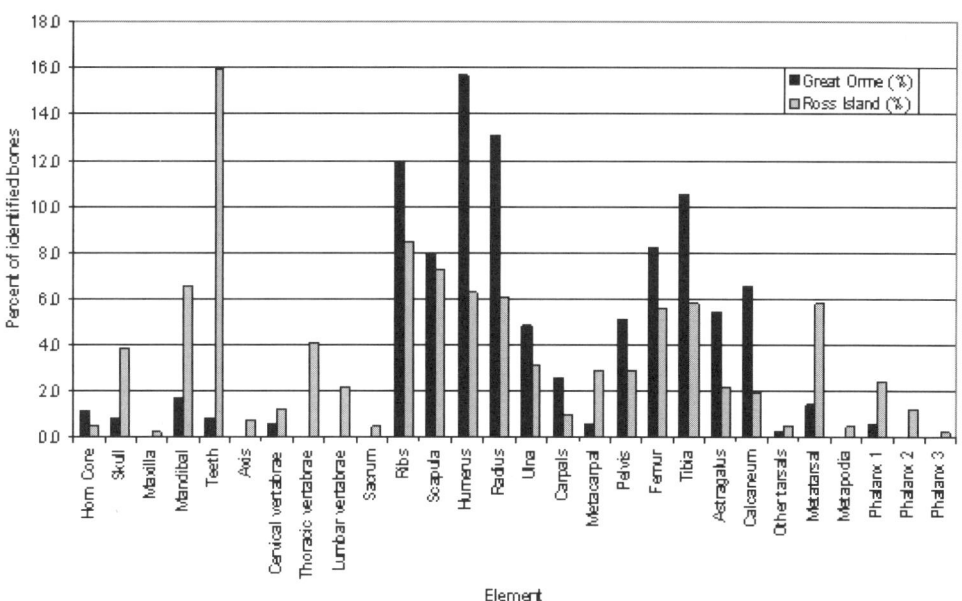

Figure 6.3. Comparative graph representing cattle skeletal fragments for Ross Island and Great Orme Mines. (Ross Island information sourced: Van Wijngaarden-Bakker 2004, 367)

Other archaeological findings can shed light on the environment on the Great Orme in the Bronze Age and the dietary habits of the miners. It has not yet been possible to obtain any archaeobotanical remains from the site; however, analysis of charred remains at Pentrwyn, a Bronze Age smelting site about two kilometres from the mine, showed emmer wheat, hazelnuts and other commonly consumed products during this time (Website 2). This site also revealed limpet and winkle shells and fish bones amongst the usual domestic debris. This contrasts markedly with the findings of food refuse at the mine and suggests that either the diet varied between the activity of mining and that of smelting copper, or the people involved in these activities were different.

Initial comparisons with other mining sites suggest that the survival of material at Great Orme is exceptional. Few copper mine sites have yielded more than a handful of faunal remains due to their acidity, so this assemblage may shed light on the gaps in evidence for Bronze Age mining activity elsewhere. Preliminary analysis of the bone from Great Orme compared to Ross Island, an Irish contemporary copper mine site, suggest a completely different pattern of faunal assemblage (Figure 6.3). Whereas Ross Island bone appear to represent whole animals brought in as a 'walking larder' (Van Wijngaarden-Bakker 2004, 370) the Great Orme assemblage suggest manageable portions brought to the site. By comparison to the Great Orme assemblage, Ross Island also yielded a higher frequency of metapodia and deer antler, as did Grimes Graves in Norfolk (Clutton-Brock 1984, 9). These robust elements are suitable for picking at the ore but perhaps they were considered unnecessary at Great Orme where the preferred method of mining appears to have been pounding with stone hammers and scraping with bone tools.

Conclusions

Most of the Great Orme assemblage represents food refuse and the quantity and nature of the faunal remains suggest that the food brought to the site was of sufficient quality to feed the miners and to provide them with utensils to carry out their work.

Workers in Wales during more recent times often combined fishing and mining; both activities carried an air of danger which led the participants to hold strong beliefs and surround each occupation with rituals (Davies 1971, 2). This does not appear to be the case for these miners in the Bronze Age; the people working at the site ignored most of the marine, coastal and hunted resources. Perhaps they felt that fish was not a suitable meal for when they were underground, maybe it was even taboo. It is possible that some of the bone refuse was regarded as ritual closing deposits for the underworld; this would be consistent with evidence from ethnographic and historical sources about ritual activity in mines.

The faunal remains from the Great Orme mines display a pattern of regimented and organized behaviour which is in keeping with all other visible aspects of the Bronze Age mining operation so far. Archaeological evidence of Bronze Age activity in Britain generally suggests the capacity for mass organization of people towards common goals, whether it was erecting stone monuments in Wessex or driving huge herds of livestock over the Fens (Pryor 2006, 113). The Great Orme Mine is a clear case for demonstrating it was happening in more Northern areas of Britain too. It has been suggested that the Bronze Age hosted societies that fuelled their conspicuous consumption by an agricultural surplus (Pryor 2006, 143). If copper was the driving force of the Bronze Age, then its miners held a crucial position in the trading network of the country and needed sustaining on a massive scale. A site of this nature must have had considerable standing during the period, therefore the creation of new data for this site should have implications for the overall picture of Bronze Age life in Britain and social and trading networks in prehistoric Europe.

The faunal remains are also a tool with which future studies can compare this industrial site to domestic occupation elsewhere; they also help alleviate the bias in data for this period from southern British sites. This study has shown the considerable potential of the faunal material at Great Orme; however, to gain a holistic understanding of Bronze Age mining at Great Orme other aspects of the site also need investigation, such as the charcoal deposits and human remains.

References

Barber, M. 2003. *Bronze and the Bronze Age, Metalwork and Society in Britain c.2500–800BC* (London).
Beecroft, S. 2005. *Evidence of Ritual Activity at the Great Orme*, Llandudno (Unpublished MA Thesis, University of Liverpool).
Bradley, R. 2000. *An Archaeology of Natural Places* (London).
Clutton-Brock, J. 1984. *Excavations at Grimes Graves, Norfolk, 1927–1976, Fascicule 1, Neolithic Antler Pick* (London).
Davies, L. 1971. 'Aspects of mining folklore in Wales', *Folk Life* **9**, 79–106.
Gravett, T. and Jowett, H. 1997. *Discovering the Great Orme* (Conwy).
Hamilton-Dyer, S. 1990. *Animal Bones from the Excavations at the Great Orme, Llandudno 1976–1989* (Southampton).
Jovanović, B. 1980. 'Primary copper mining and the production of copper', in Craddock, P. (ed.) *Scientific Studies in Early Mining and Extractive Metallurgy* (London), 31–40.
Lewis, C.A. 1996. *Prehistoric Mining at the Great Orme: Criteria for the Identification of Early Mining* (Unpublished MPhil Thesis, University of Wales, Bangor).
Outram, A.K. 2002. 'Bone fracture and within-bone nutrients: an experimentally based method for investigating levels of marrow extraction', in Miracle, P. and Milner, N. (eds) *Consuming Passions and Patterns of Consumption* (Cambridge), 51–64.
Palmer, J.D. 2001. *Animal Wisdom* (London).
Pryor, F. 2003. *Britain BC* (London).
Pryor, F. 2006. *Farmers in Prehistoric Britain* (Gloucestershire).
Timberlake, S. 2003. *Excavations on Copa Hill, Cwmystwyth (1986–1999); An Early Bronze Age copper mine within the uplands of Central Wales* (Oxford).
Van Wijngaarden-Bakker, L.H. 2004. 'The animal remains', in O'Brien, W. (ed.) *Ross Island: Mining, Metal and Society in Early Ireland* (Galway), 367–86.
Wager, E. 2002. *The Character and Context of Bronze Age Mining on the Great Orme, North Wales, UK* (Unpublished PhD Thesis, University of Sheffield).

Website 1. http://www.britarch.ac.uk/ba/ba58/news.shtml#inbrief
Website 2. http://www.ancient-arts.org/projects.htm

An Isotopic Approach to Diet in Medieval Spain

Michelle Mundee,
University of Durham

Medieval Spain presents a unique opportunity to examine the archaeology of a multi-faith society, first under Muslim and later under Christian rule. Unlike other areas of Europe, Spain has been neglected in archaeological studies of medieval diet. This paper presents a preliminary case study of a Christian population in Jaca, north-east Spain. Stable carbon ($\delta^{13}C$) and nitrogen ($\delta^{15}N$) isotope ratios were measured in adult human bone collagen. Initial results suggest that the majority of Christians in the city in the thirteenth to fifteenth centuries AD consumed similar foodstuffs to Muslims in the nearby urban centre of Zaragoza two centuries before. Possible migrants have been identified with a significant proportion of C_4 in their diet, as opposed to the C_3-based diet of the majority. Data from contemporaneous animal bone is essential to understand further trends observed in this preliminary study.

Background

Multi-faith societies existed around the Mediterranean during the medieval period, most notably in urban, mercantile communities in Spain. Christians, Muslims and Jews co-existed under Muslim rule after the Arab conquest in the eighth century AD (Collins 1989). Christian rule followed the Reconquista, when Muslim territory was gradually re-conquered over the course of two to three centuries, gaining particular momentum after the twelfth century AD (Barton 2004). Only in 1492 did Granada, the last remaining Muslim stronghold, surrender. The same year, Jews were expelled from Spain (Anderson 2002, 97–98). Of particular interest here is that Moriscos, Muslims who had converted to Christianity, were only expelled from Spain in 1609 (Anderson 2002, 116).

The aim of this research is to assess differences in diet between individuals and between faith communities, and to analyse those differences under differing political control over an extended time period. Much of the current understanding of diet in medieval Iberia is based on indirect written historical sources (e.g. Adamson 2004; Garcia Sanchez 2002); there is a paucity of published archaeological evidence from botanical and zooarchaeological studies. The technique used here to reconstruct diet is isotopic analysis, which provides a direct method for elucidating diet at the level of the individual. Specifically, carbon ($\delta^{13}C$) and nitrogen ($\delta^{15}N$) isotope ratios from Christian and Muslim bone collagen have been utilized to explore differences in diet within a transect of north-east Spain, from the Pyrenees to the coast. Both Christian and Muslim

An Isotopic Approach to Diet in Medieval Spain

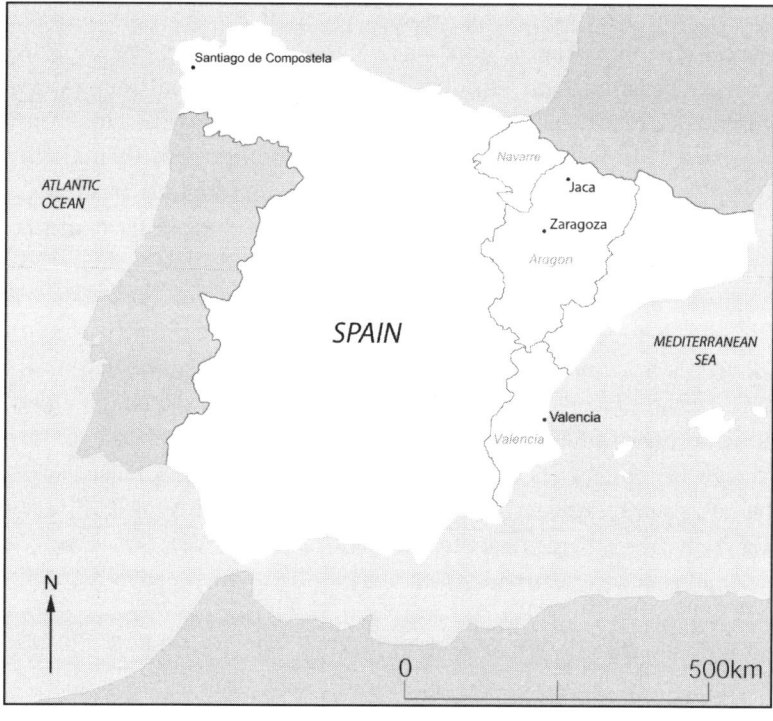

Figure 7.1. Map of Spain showing sites mentioned in the text.

individuals have been sampled from recent, well recorded and dated archaeological excavations from six sites in the regional autonomous communities of Aragon, Valencia and Navarra which include Zaragoza and Valencia, two major medieval cities. These sites have a collective date range between the tenth and sixteenth centuries AD. This paper presents the results of a case study from the Christian urban centre of Jaca.

Stable isotopic analysis

Stable isotope analysis is a well-established technique which has been used for over 30 years to reconstruct the diet of archaeological populations (for recent general reviews of isotopic techniques in archaeology see Sealy 2001 and Katzenberg 2000). The technique is based on the principle that stable isotopes of carbon and nitrogen are incorporated into human and animal body tissues from the foods consumed during their lifetime, and this dietary signature persists in the skeletal tissues recovered from an archaeological site. Bone is renewed and replaced over 10–30 years throughout an individual's life and therefore gives information about an approximate long-term average diet of an individual before death (Ambrose 1993, 110). Collagen, the most abundant protein within bone, is routinely extracted and analysed in dietary studies and is thought to reflect the main sources of protein in the diet rather than the diet as a whole (Ambrose and Norr 1993).

Carbon isotope ratios (expressed as $\delta^{13}C$ when referred to a standard) are used to distinguish between terrestrial and marine foods (Chisholm *et al.* 1982) as well as between C_3 and C_4 plants, which use different photosynthetic pathways (Van der Merwe and Vogel 1978). C_3 plants include the majority of trees and shrubs in temperate zones such as north-west Europe and northern Spain, including crops such as wheat, barley and oats. C_4 plants grow in more arid environments and include tropical grasses such as millet, sugar cane and sorghum (Ambrose 1993, 86). These latter plants are thought to have been potentially important crops in Muslim Spain, unlike the rest of medieval Christian Europe, where C_3 crops were commonly cultivated (Glick 2005, 76–78).

The nitrogen isotope ratio ($\delta^{15}N$, when referred to a standard) of animal tissues increases with each trophic level. Therefore, by measuring $\delta^{15}N$ values in bone, identification of herbivores, omnivores and carnivores becomes possible in both marine and terrestrial ecosystems (Bocherens and Drucker 2003; Schoeninger and DeNiro 1984). Nitrogen isotope values can also be used to distinguish a reliance on marine or terrestrial foods, since marine resources tend to have higher $\delta^{15}N$ values due to the longer lengths of aquatic food chains (Schoeninger and DeNiro 1984). Stable isotope ratios of carbon and nitrogen, however, cannot be used to distinguish between consumption of different animal products – meat and milk cannot be distinguished isotopically. Thus, whether an individual gained their protein through the consumption of meat or dairy products cannot be ascertained (O'Connell and Hedges 1999).

Isotopic studies of medieval populations

This study represents the first application of isotopic techniques to medieval populations from the Spanish mainland. Previous isotopic research into the medieval diet has focused on northern Europe with studies for example in Belgium (Polet and Katzenberg 2003), England (Lakin 2008; Müldner and Richards 2005; 2007) and France (Herrscher *et al.* 2001). In general, there has been a concordance between isotopic studies of diet focusing on medieval populations and available historical and archaeological records. Isotopic evidence from English sites such as York, has identified a significant shift in diet to higher $\delta^{15}N$ values, suggesting an increase in consumption of marine resources, which may be a result of fasting laws introduced by the Church and the growth of urban centres from around the eleventh century AD (Müldner and Richards 2005; 2007). Isotopic studies of medieval populations from the Mediterranean, however, have been limited. Bourbou and Richards (2007) carried out research on human remains from medieval Greece which revealed that populations had a predominantly C_3 diet, including animal sources with a small input from marine resources. Results from a recent study from Italy (Salamon *et al.* 2008) conducted on individuals from two inland populations dating to the seventh and fifteenth centuries AD seem to reflect the same trend for increased consumption of marine resources during the later medieval period, as identified on English sites.

Historical evidence for Christian diet in medieval Spain

The traditional view of the Mediterranean diet emphasizes the essential triad of wheat, wine and olives (Braudel 1966, 236), although the important role of animal products must also be taken into account. Wheat may have been more of a high-status grain; the lower strata of society would have probably eaten more rye and barley or mixed-grain bread (Glick 2005, 91). Fruit and vegetables would have also played an important part in the diet; but, as they are low in protein, they cannot be distinguished from other C_3 crops using isotopic analysis. Other important crops consumed include pulses and legumes (Horden and Purcell 2000, 203). Fish caught from the Mediterranean and the Atlantic and freshwater lakes and rivers would have been available to most strata of society. Fish was preserved in a number of ways during the medieval period and therefore could be traded over long distances inland (Anderson 2002, 185). Meat such as lamb, goat, pork, chicken, game and beef would have been available to some; however, eggs and dairy products such as cheese and milk would have been consumed more often by the poorer classes (Anderson 2002, 187).

Case study: Jaca

Jaca lies in northern Aragon near the modern-day border with France. Lying so far north, the city was only briefly occupied by the Muslims, and certainly was under Christian control before the ninth century AD, though the exact date of re-conquest is unknown (Buesa Conde 2004). During the later Middle Ages, Jaca was an important city. It was the capital of the Christian kingdom of Aragon until 1097. It lay on important travel and trade routes between Zaragoza and southern France as well as a major pilgrimage route to Santiago de Compostela (Buesa Conde 2004). Pilgrims to Santiago were identified among the burials excavated at the site of Plaza Biscós in Jaca by the placement of scallop shells, the symbol of St James, with the body (Justes 2006). One individual was buried with three shells, indicating multiple pilgrimages (Justes 2006). Individuals sampled from this site will characterize a Christian diet in northern Spain that would not have been greatly influenced by Muslim political control.

Materials and methods

Twenty-seven individuals dating to the thirteenth to fifteenth centuries AD were sampled from the Christian cemetery of Plaza Biscós in Jaca. Samples of rib (~200mg) were selected from complete burials that I determined to be skeletally adult. Although faunal samples were also taken from excavations in nearby Huesca, results are pending. Therefore, the dataset here lacks a faunal baseline. A faunal baseline would enable the human data to be better understood within the isotopic variation of the local environment and available foodstuffs. Collagen extraction followed the standard method outlined in Richards and Hedges (1999) with an additional filtration step (Brown *et al.* 1988) to further 'purify' the collagen extract. The prepared collagen was analysed at the Stable Isotope Facility at the University of Alaska Fairbanks's Water

& Environmental Research Center, USA, using a continuous-flow Delta+XP isotope ratio mass spectrometer interfaced with a Costech ECS 4010 elemental analyzer. Stable isotope ratios were reported in δ notation as parts per thousand or per mill (‰) deviation from the international standards PDB (carbon) and Air (nitrogen). Typically, instrument precision is <0.2 per mill for both $\delta^{13}C$ and $\delta^{15}N$. Samples were run in duplicate and the average of the two runs for each sample is presented here. Collagen preservation was generally good, with two samples failing to yield sufficient collagen and only one sample failing to fall within the accepted range of the C:N ratio collagen quality indicator (Van Klinken 1999). These samples are not considered here.

Results

In the absence of contemporaneous faunal data, individuals from Jaca were plotted against the mean of 37 adult Muslims of similar social status from the nearby urban centre of Zaragoza dating to the tenth to twelfth centuries (see Figure 7.2). The mean of $\delta^{13}C$ values for Jaca is -18.35 ±1.2 per mill (1σ). A group of four individuals clearly, on the graph, do not plot with the majority (circled in Figure 7.2), with higher $\delta^{13}C$ values within the range of -17.0 to -15.3 per mill. There are also two further individuals who can be described as intermediate between the two different groups in terms of their $\delta^{13}C$

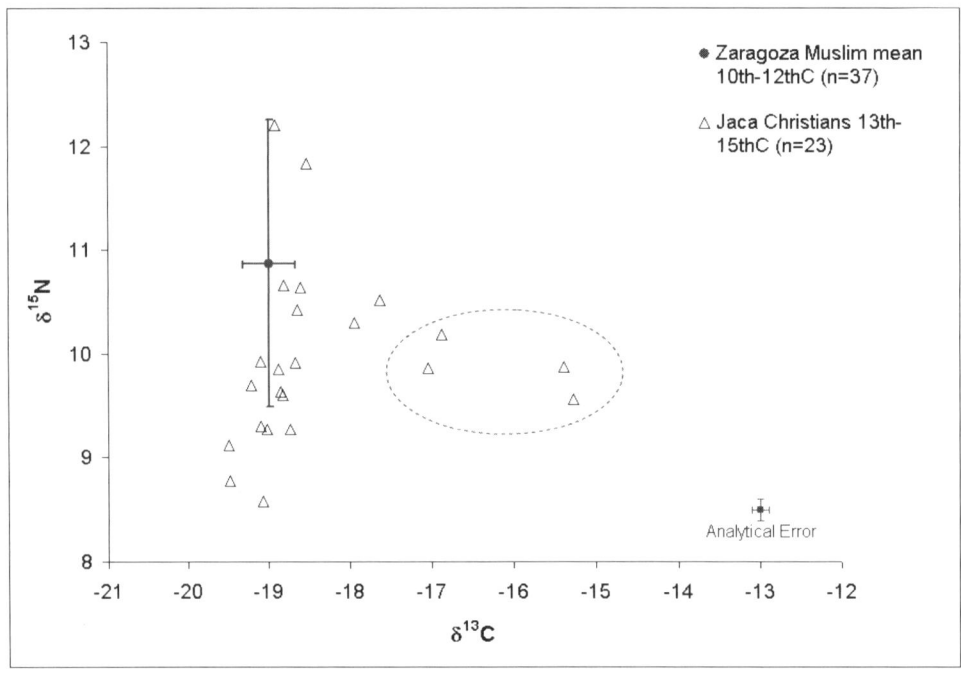

Figure 7.2. Scatter plot of $\delta^{13}C$ and $\delta^{15}N$ values for Christians from Jaca in comparison with the mean for Muslims in Zaragoza (mean ± 1σ). Possible migrants are circled (source: Mundee in prep.).

values. The mean of $\delta^{15}N$ values from Jaca is 9.96 ±0.9 per mill, with most individuals plotting within the range of 8.6–10.6 per mill, although two outliers can be identified demonstrating significant enrichment in ^{15}N.

Discussion

The majority of individuals from Jaca plot closely with Muslims from Zaragoza, especially in terms of their $\delta^{13}C$ values, which indicate a mainly C_3, terrestrial-based diet. It may be expected that Muslims would plot differently to Christians due to differing dietary laws, with Muslims consuming less ^{15}N rich protein from omnivorous domesticates such as pork. However, differences are not observed in the isotopic evidence presented here.

The $\delta^{15}N$ values of both populations are relatively high, which suggests that their dietary protein derived mainly from animal sources such as dairy products and meat. The wide range in nitrogen exhibited by samples from Jaca (3.6 per mill) is similar to the trend seen in historic-period populations from elsewhere (Müldner and Richards 2005, 2007; Bourbou and Richards 2007). This range in values may reflect the consumption of varying amounts of fish, possibly deriving from freshwater, riverine resources which would have been readily available from the River Aragon which runs through Jaca. In particular, the two individuals with higher $\delta^{15}N$ values coupled with a terrestrial carbon signature may have been eating more terrestrial/freshwater protein than the majority. Isotopic data for fish bones from this site would clarify this suggestion, and the analysis of other animal remains would also help to prove whether these apparent variations reflect differences in human diet or simply local variation in nitrogen isotopes in the available foodstuffs.

The markedly high $\delta^{13}C$ values of four isolated individuals indicate a C_4 contribution to their diet. A number of hypotheses may explain their difference in diet. It may be that they represent a small group of local people who had a different diet to the rest of the population or that they chose to fodder the animals they consumed on C_4 foodstuffs such as millet. Isotopic results from local faunal remains could confirm this. Given that they represent a relatively small proportion of the number of individuals analysed, it may be more likely that they are outsiders who originated from elsewhere. Hardy, arid-loving C_4 crops are thought to have been cultivated in Muslim Spain (Constable 1994, 162) and sorghum is believed to have been brought over to al-Andalus from North Africa (Glick 2005, 76). It has been suggested that wheat, a C_3 crop, was not held in high regard and that the good health of the Andalusis, particularly those from rural areas, could be attributed to 'their spartan diet of sorghum and olive oil,' (Ibn Khaldūn 1958, cited by Glick 2005, 78). The individuals in the sample above may therefore have originated from further south in Spain. In that case, they were possibly Mozarabs, Christians under Muslim rule, who had migrated and settled in the Christian north. This suggestion is further supported by their wide range in $\delta^{13}C$ values which is similar to individuals previously published from ancient North Africa where C_4 crops were also available (Thompson *et al.* 2008). Alternatively, these individuals may be unidentified pilgrims to Santiago buried without scallop shells. However, Santiago de Compostela lies on the north-west tip of Spain and it is inherently unlikely that a pilgrim from the south would have travelled a route through Jaca to the north-east. A more likely explanation therefore is that the individuals may represent merchants or travellers making their way north into France.

The two individuals with $\delta^{13}C$ values that lie between the majority and the isolated group may also be immigrants who had settled in Jaca for a number of years, since their average bone collagen isotope signature is seen to be shifting towards the local dietary signal of the majority sampled.

Furthermore, migrants could possibly be identified by tracing their life histories through different body tissues such as tooth dentine as it does not undergo significant modelling like bone and therefore reflects the diet consumed during its formation in childhood (Sealy *et al.* 1995). Strontium and oxygen isotopes in tooth enamel may also establish whether the individuals were local to the area (Sealy 2001). However, further analysis on other surviving archaeological biological tissues is currently beyond the scope of this exploratory case study. Undoubtedly, the results from animal bone data will significantly aid the interpretation of these results.

Conclusions

Initial results suggest that the Christian diet in Jaca between the thirteenth and fifteenth centuries AD was similar to that found at Muslim sites in northern Spain two centuries earlier. Similar types of foodstuffs, a C_3 based diet with varying amounts of marine/aquatic protein, were therefore likely to have been eaten at these sites. These findings fit with other studies of later medieval Mediterranean populations (Salamon *et al.* 2008; Bourbou and Richards 2007). Possible migrants have also been identified at Jaca due to a significant proportion of C_4 in their diet and their isotopic signature being substantially different from the local population. These individuals may represent travellers or merchants from other regions of Spain or further afield where C_4 crops are cultivated, or local individuals with a C_4 enriched diet. It must be stressed that the results are provisional: the integration of faunal results with the data will further the understanding of the trends outlined here.

The case study presented here demonstrates the utility of isotopic techniques in elucidating diet at the individual level and highlights the potential of this technique to reveal trends in diet within medieval Spain. Further work will focus on enlarging the dataset to allow a more in-depth study of diet across the whole sampled region of north-east Spain with the integration of faunal results.

An Isotopic Approach to Diet in Medieval Spain

Acknowledgements

Many thanks to Dr Christopher Gerrard, Dr Alejandra Gutierrez and Dr Andrew Millard (Durham University); all those who facilitated my sample collection in Spain, specifically Julia Justes and the Provincial Museum of Huesca and also the Alaska Stable Isotope Facility for isotopic analysis. This research was funded by the AHRC with contributions from a Durham Doctoral Fellowship.

References

Adamson, M.W. 2004. *Food in Medieval Times* (Westport CT), 115–124.

Ambrose, S.H. 1993. 'Isotopic analysis of palaeodiets: methodological and interpretative considerations', in Sandford, M.K. (ed.) *Investigations of Ancient Human Tissue: Chemical Analyses in Anthropology* (Langthorne), 59–130.

Ambrose, S.H. and Norr, L. 1993. 'Experimental evidence for the relationship of the carbon isotope ratios of whole diet and dietary protein to those of bone collagen and carbonate', in Lambert, J.B. and Grupe, G. (eds) *Prehistoric Human Bone: Archaeology at the Molecular Level* (Berlin), 1–37.

Anderson, J.M. 2002. *Daily Life During the Spanish Inquisition* (Westport CT).

Barton, S. 2004. *A History of Spain* (Basingstoke).

Bocherens, H. and Drucker, D. 2003. 'Trophic level enrichment of carbon and nitrogen in bone collagen: case studies from recent and terrestrial ecosystems', *International Journal of Osteoarchaeology* 13, 46–53.

Bourbou, C and Richards, M.P. 2007. 'The Middle Byzantine menu: palaeodietary information from isotopic analysis of humans and fauna from Kastella, Crete', *International Journal of Osteoarchaeology* 17, 63–72.

Braudel, F. 1966. *The Mediterranean and the Mediterranean World in the Age of Philip II*, 2 vols. (New York).

Brown, T.A., Nelson, D.E., Vogel, J.S. and Southon, J.R. 1988. 'Improved collagen extraction by modified longin method', *Radiocarbon* 30, 171–7.

Buesca Conde, D.J. 2004 'Jaca, primera capital del Reino de Aragón', in Gonzáles, J.L.O. and Lanaspa, S.S. (eds) *Comarca de la Jacetania* (Diputación General de Aragón), 73–8.

Chisholm, B.S., Nelson, D.E and Schwarcz, H.P. 1982. 'Stable carbon isotope ratios as a measure of marine versus terrestrial protein in ancient diets', *Science* 216, 1131–2.

Collins, R. 1989. *The Arab Conquest of Spain* (Oxford).

Constable, O.R. 1994. *Trade and Traders in Muslim Spain* (Cambridge).

Garcia Sanchez, E. 2002. 'Dietic aspects of food in al-Andalus', in Waines, D (ed.) *Patterns of Everyday Life* (Aldershot), 275–88.

Glick, T.F. 2005. *Islamic and Christian Spain in the Early Middle Ages* (Leiden, Boston).

Herrscher, E., Bocherens, H., Valentin, F. and Colardelle, R. 2001. 'Comportements alimentaires au Moyen Âge à Grenoble: application de la biogéochimie isotopique à la nécropole Saint-Laurent (XIIIe–XVe siècles, Isère, France)', *C.R. Acad. Sci. Paris, Sciences de la vie / Life Sciences* 324, 479–87.

Horden, P. and Purcell, N. 2000. *The Corrupting Sea: A Study of Mediterranean History* (Oxford).

Ibn Khaldūn (trans. Franz Rosenthal) 1958. *The Muqaddimah: An Introduction to History* (New York).

Justes, J. 2006. *Plaza Biscós, Jaca Expediente: 26/03/06* (Unpublished Excavation Report, Huesca).

Katzenberg, M.A. 2000. 'Stable isotope analysis: a tool for studying past diet, demography and life history', in Katzenberg, M.A. and Saunders, S.R. (eds) *The Biological Anthropology of the Human Skeleton* (New York), 305–27.

Lakin, K. 2008. 'Medieval diet: evidence for a London signature?', in Baker, S., Allen, M., Middle, S. and Poole, K. (eds.) *Food and Drink in Archaeology 1* (Totnes), 65–72.

Müldner, G. and Richards, M.P. 2005. 'Fast or feast: reconstructing diet in later medieval England by stable isotope analysis', *Journal of Archaeological Science* 32, 39–48.

Müldner, G. and Richards, M.P. 2007. 'Stable isotope evidence for 1500 years of diet at the city of York, UK', *American Journal of Physical Anthropology* **133**, 682–97.

Mundee, M.M. in prep. *An isotopic approach to diet within the multi-faith society of medieval Spain* (PhD Thesis, Durham University).

O'Connell, T.C. and Hedges, R.E.M. 1999. 'Investigations into the effect of diet on modern human hair isotopic values', *American Journal of Physical Anthropology* **108**, 409–25.

Polet, C. and Katzenberg, M.A. 2003.' Reconstruction of the diet in a medieval monastic community from the coast of Belgium', *Journal of Archaeological Science* **30**, 525–33.

Richards, M.P. and Hedges, R.E.M. 1999. 'Stable isotope evidence for similarities in the types of marine foods used by the late Mesolithic humans at sites along the Atlantic coast of Europe', *Journal of Archaeological Science* **26**, 717–22.

Salamon, M., Coppa, A., McCormick, M., Rubini, M., Vargiu, R. and Tuross, N. 2008. 'The consilience of historical and isotopic approaches in reconstructing the medieval Mediterranean diet', *Journal of Archaeological Science* **35**, 1667–72.

Schoeninger, M.J. and DeNiro, M.J. 1984. 'Stable nitrogen and carbon isotopic composition of bone collagen from marine and terrestrial animals', *Geochimica et Cosmochimica Acta* **48**, 625–39.

Sealy, J. 2001. 'Body tissue chemistry and palaeodiet', in Brothwell, D.R.and Pollard, A.M. (eds) *Handbook of Archaeological Science* (Chichester), 269–79.

Sealy, J., Armstrong, R. and Schrire, C. 1995. 'Beyond lifetime averages: tracing life histories through isotopic analysis of different calcified tissues from archaeological human skeletons', *Antiquity* **69**, 290–300.

Thompson, A.H., Chaix, L. and Richards, M.P. 2008. 'Stable isotopes and diet at ancient Kerma, Upper Nubia (Sudan)', *Journal of Archaeological Science* **35**, 376–87.

Van Klinken, G.J. 1999. 'Bone collagen quality indicators for palaeodietary and radiocarbon measurements', *Journal of Archeological Science* **26**, 687–995.

Van der Merwe, N.J. and Vogel, J.C. 1978. '^{13}C content of human collagen as a measure of prehistoric diet in Woodland North America', *Nature* **276**, 815–6.

The Ritualization of Eating and Drinking: Politics, Religion and Food Consumption in Pre-Roman Veneto, Italy

Elisa Perego,
University College London

Anthropology and archaeology have long recognized the importance of eating and drinking as powerful metaphors and practices employed to negotiate socio-political and economic dynamics (Appadurai 1981; Bray 2003; Dietler and Hayden 2001; Goody 1982). This paper explores how the ceremonial consumption of food and beverages was reflected in the ritual manipulation of culinary implements in pre-Roman Veneto. The Veneti flourished in north-eastern Italy in the first millennium BC. Their society, based since the ninth century BC on the affiliation between kin-group members, over the following four centuries evolved towards a more articulated organization of extended elite families and their subordinates. From the sixth century, a deeper interaction with Celts, Etruscans and Greeks, as well as internal growth, were among the factors which led to urbanization, the adoption of writing and more structured forms of cult in sanctuaries (Capuis 2004). Approximately 15 cult places are known from different Venetic localities, ranging from peak sacred sites to sanctuaries surrounding the settlement of Este. At these sites (e.g. Lagole, San Pietro Montagnon, Este Meggiaro and Baratella, and Villa di Villa) a great variety of ritual practices is observed such as animal sacrifice, banqueting, initiations, intentional breakage of objects, divination and offering of ornaments and bronze plaques (Gorini and Mastrocinque 2005; Ruta Serafini 2002). Venetic funerary ritual was complex, involving secondary burial, ideological construction of the deceased's identity and deliberate mixing of bones and grave goods between the members of the same tomb. Cremation was the main funerary ritual, but inhumation was also practised. Grave goods included ornaments, tools, vessels, food and weapons (Chieco Bianchi and Calzavara Capuis 1985; 2006). The tomb's structure could vary from stone and wooden containers to ceramic vessels and pits. Cremation graves were generally covered by pyre debris and a tumulus. Tombs belonging to the same family/clan were placed adjacent to each other and included in collective tumuli. Marginal people were disposed of in pits or inhumed along the tumulus edge, while the uppermost elites were buried in grand multiple tombs located in the middle of the collective mounds (Balista and Ruta Serafini 1998).

Information on Venetic alimentary habits is provided by food remains excavated in sanctuaries, tombs and settlements. The food consumed included meat, fowl, fish, shellfish, cereals, legumes and fruits (Motella De Carlo 2002; Ruta Serafini and Sainati

2002, 222; Vitri 1996, 404). This evidence, however, is still too fragmentary to allow us to distinguish everyday from ritual cuisine, to recognize dietary taboos or to determine social change from dining practices. Nonetheless, the fact that the Veneti ascribed a fundamental importance to specific dining practices can be inferred from the ritual manipulation of culinary implements interred in graves, sanctuaries and under the house floor. A particular emphasis was given to the ritual consumption of alcohol, with the partial integration of foreign cultural models (e.g. the Greek symposium) into the local elites' lifestyle, and the possible exclusion of non-elite social segments from this form of commensality.

Sanctuaries

Consumption of food and drink was one of the main aspects of Venetic religious practice, as testified by the large quantity of animal bones, vegetal remains and culinary implements excavated in sacred sites (Dammer 2002a; Fiore and Tagliacozzo 2002; Gregnanin 2002). The typology of culinary equipment and the analysis of organic remains provide information on the rituals performed in different sanctuaries and on the involvement of different social groups. The elites' involvement in the ritual practice at the main Venetic sacred sites is testified by the relative abundance of prestige offerings such as ornaments, iconic bronze plaques, fine pottery and bronze vessels (e.g. Ruta Serafini and Sainati 2002). An exception is probably offered by the sanctuary of San Pietro Montagnon (Padua), where the presence of a huge quantity of rough ceramics alongside more prestigious offerings suggests the participation of both elite and non-elite social segments (Dammer 2002b).

The offerings for the deity included selected animal bones, vegetal portions and animals burned on ritual fires, and entire carcasses including pig foetuses and pregnant sows buried untouched (Dammer 2002a, 253; Fiore and Tagliacozzo 2002). I would suggest that burning, which had perhaps its counterpart in funerary cremation, was employed to allow the offering to change its status and be consumed by the god. This hypothesis is strengthened by the fact that holocausts were extended even to metal figurines of horses burned instead of the real animal (Dammer 2002b, 302). In this case burning was clearly not intended to render the offering edible for the worshippers, but rather to negotiate how the gift was made available to the deity. The practice of drinking in honour of the god is testified by the deposition of cups inscribed with the worshipper's and the deity's name (Tirelli 2002, 312). The deliberate breakage of culinary implements and ritual paraphernalia was widely diffused (Bonomi 2003, 48; Tirelli 2002, 315) and perhaps motivated by the desire to free the 'soul' of the offering. Other explanations, however, are possible. Ritual paraphernalia may have been destroyed when considered polluted, dangerous or sacred – and thus unemployable after the ceremony. When culinary vessels were interred deliberately incomplete (Gregnanin 2002, 165), fragmentation (*sensu* Chapman and Gaydarska 2007) may have allowed the redistribution of fragments, retained by the worshippers as mementos of the ceremony or employed in other rituals.

The Ritualization of Eating and Drinking

Graves

Food and culinary equipment were offered to the dead both on the pyre and in the grave (Motella De Carlo 1998, 60; Ruta Serafini 1990, 44–45, 138). The complete dining set placed in the tomb included a wide range of bronze and ceramic implements for food preparation and consumption (Chieco Bianchi 1987; Chieco Bianchi and Calzavara Capuis 1985; 2006). Bowls of different kinds were buried with the meal for the dead, while beverages were contained in bigger vessels (*situlae*). Cups, beakers and, later, jugs were used to drink from and to pour liquids, respectively. Firedogs may have alluded to the custody of the domestic fireplace, while spits were used to roast meat. *Spatulae* (slices) were probably employed to cut and offer soft food. More difficult to understand is the value of axes and knives, which may have been weapons, ritual items and/or culinary implements related to meat butchering (e.g. Ruta Serafini 2004, 281). Strainers were present in a few tombs of significant wealth possibly to emphasize the role of the aristocrat in charge of the beverage preparation. Evidence from late prehistoric Italy and the Veneto suggests that the task of filtering alcohol from aromatic spices may have been performed by elite individuals who, by taking control of precious intoxicants, reaffirmed their power over subordinates at the ritual banquet (Iaia 2006, 106). Rarely, however, was the entire assemblage described above buried in a single tomb. Differences in the composition of the service were possibly due to the sex, age and rank of the deceased. The uppermost elites, for example, were endowed with a wealth of bronze vessels and fine pottery, while low-ranking children were given just a minimal provision. However, since Venetic tombs were often re-opened to accommodate more individuals, and grave goods were manipulated, a clear association between any specific dead and its own service is precisely detectable only in the case of single graves.

The ritualization of eating and drinking practices in funerary contexts was reinforced by the placing of laminated culinary implements and ritually broken vessels in tombs (e.g. Chieco Bianchi and Calzavara Capuis 1985, 246–7; 2006, 262). Laminated items such as spits and knives were clearly not intended for real use and alluded to the ritual banquet consumed for the dead. The interment of broken drinking vessels in tomb tumuli is probably evidence of libations performed when the grave was closed (e.g. Chieco Bianco and Calzavara Capuis 1985, 300–311). The deposition of incomplete vessels inside the grave suggests that, as proposed by Chapman and Gaydarska (2007) for the prehistoric Balkans, fragments of ritually-charged implements may have been retained in the world of the living as mementos of the dead and/or to be employed in other ceremonies. This is particularly evident when fragments were placed in single graves not disturbed after the first deposition (e.g. Chieco Bianchi and Calzavara Capuis 2006, 255). In these cases fragmentation did not derive from further manipulation and involuntary breakage of grave goods but was clearly intended as a meaningful and deliberate practice. Another element which emphasized the symbolic contiguity between funerary rituals and eating practices was the use of culinary vessels as urns. In elite tomb Este Ricovero 232, for example, the bronze urns had been used to cook food before deposition, as testified by the traces of soot still present in the vessels (Chieco Bianchi and Calzavara Capuis 1985, 273). The adoption of culinary vessels as burial urns suggests that human remains may have been conceived as metaphorical food, with the possibility, for the mourners, to elaborate symbolic links between selected foods and the dead. Further, as noted by Oestigaard (2000) for Iron Age Scandinavia, cremated (i.e. cooked) humans can be intended as alimentary offerings for the deity. The hypothesis is intriguing, since, as shown above, in Venetic sanctuaries burning may have been employed to allow the offering to reach the deity. This interpretation, which requires further elaboration and a more in-depth study of inhumation practices, suggests that cremation, as well as the adoption of more or less prestigious culinary vessels as urns, may have been means through which power was maintained and negotiated by allowing certain individuals to become food for the deity and achieve special status after death.

Houses

Recent excavations have provided rich information on Venetic building techniques (Ruta Serafini 2003). Houses were built in timber covered with clay, arranged in accurately planned quarters and supplied with fireplaces, cisterns and gullies. Foundation rituals included the deposition of offerings under the floor. In such occasions, the interment of luxurious implements for food and wine consumption may have alluded to the ritualization of formal dining habits. The wealth of the bronze vessels and drinking cups unearthed under the house floor and their similarity with examples found in elite graves suggests that caches were interred by the members of privileged social classes. The deposit excavated in Via Battisti at Padua, for instance, included 20 ceramic vessels and a set of metal instruments for serving wine and food preparation (Bianco *et al.* 1998, 107–37). The most prestigious item, a *skyphos* cup imitating vessels produced in Campania, south Italy, recalled in its typology Attic models employed at the Greek symposium. Similar wine-drinking forms, several of them produced directly in Athens, have been found in Venetic sanctuaries and wealthy graves (e.g. Bonomi 2003; Chieco Bianchi 1987). The cache's ritual value was emphasized by the reduced dimensions of several ceramic containers, perhaps not employable in everyday meals, and by the fact that the metal implements were laminated and clearly not intended for real use. The *skyphos*, moreover, was ritually broken (handle removed). Other elements of the deposit implied a direct link with religious and even magical practices. A laminated horse figurine and a bronze disk may have alluded to the mythical voyage of the sun in the sky, while two pig bones – one inscribed – were possibly used for divination. The pierced pebble can be compared with identical examples excavated in wealthy children's urns in association with amulets/ornaments, such as glass beads and cowries (e.g. Chieco Bianchi and Calzavara Capuis 2006, 227).

The Ritualization of Eating and Drinking

The power of drinking

The importance of alcoholic beverages in negotiating political power has already been emphasized (Dietler 1990). In Greece, the communal consumption of wine took the form of the symposium, a highly ritualized practice performed under the auspices of the deity, where bonds of friendship and hospitality between aristocratic males were negotiated and reinforced (Lissarrague 1990; Schuitema 2008). In Central Europe and Italy, the establishment of formal drinking practices probably took place at the beginning of the Iron Age (*c.* ninth century BC), when elaborate drinking sets started to appear in elite graves (Iaia 2006). In the Veneto, the consumption of special liquids assumed a paramount importance in the early Iron Age, although it is unclear whether the beverage consumed was wine. In tomb Este Ricovero 236, a multiple grave of exceptional ritual complexity, the male dead (the gender is conjectural) was placed in a bronze *situla* imported from continental Europe, and possibly used as a wine container before deposition. The urn also contained a bronze service composed of a second bronze container, two cups to pour liquids and three strainers. All these implements were burned on the pyre with the dead and emphasized the man's control over beverage distribution. Conversely, the numerous ceramic cups found outside the urn could refer to the funeral's participants, who, being in a subordinate position with respect to the deceased, were allowed to drink but not to manipulate the beverage (Iaia 2006, 108).

By the late sixth century, the Greeks had codified a complex repertoire of symposium equipments including vessels for mixing wine with water (*kraters*) and drinking cups such as *kylikes* and *skyphoi* (Lissarrague 1990). The exportation of wine and sympotic implements from Greece reinforced previous commercial routes which, often through Etruria, reached Central Europe, the Western Mediterranean and the Veneto (Bonomi 2003; Dietler 1990, 2–4). The acquisition of exotic drinking practices by the Veneti is demonstrated by the presence of Greek sympotic vessels in sanctuaries, settlements and elite graves (e.g. Bonomi 2003; Chieco Bianchi 1987; Ruta Serafini 2003). However, strong evidence also indicates the independence of local elites with respect to external cultural inputs. The extreme selectivity in the choice of the vessels acquired – *skyphoi* and *kylikes*, for example, but rarely *kraters* – emphasizes the careful adoption of foreign commodities into a system which was already perfectly established. The autonomy of Venetic elites is further proved by the existence of different patterns of consumption in the two main settlements of Padua and Este. In the former, the abundance of Attic vessels in wealthy settlement quarters set against their total lack in tombs probably indicates the persistence of local forms of commensality in occasion of funerary rituals. In the latter, the presence of Greek vessels in elite graves suggests the adoption of foreign drinking practices also during the funeral (Leonardi 2004, 288).

Another element of diversity between the Greek and the Venetic symposium is the active involvement of elite women in the latter, possibly due to Etruscan influence. This is testified both by the presence of sympotic vessels in luxurious female graves (e.g. Chieco Bianchi 1987) and by the iconographic motif engraved on a bronze belt-plaque found in tomb Este Carceri 48 (Frey 1969, table 28). The belt-plaque represents a symposium scene involving a man on a couch and a woman about to serve him, both of them dressed as aristocrats. The use of belt-plaques by elite women both in sanctuaries and funerary contexts (Capuis and Chieco Bianchi 2002, 238–9), and the presence of imported Greek vessels in cult places, elaborate tombs and wealthy settlement quarters demonstrate that the Venetic banquet, given ritual significance through allusions to the religious sphere and the Greek symposium, became a locus of disparity between the elite who adopted the Attic vessels imported in the Veneto, and the social segments who had a marginal role in these forms of commensality.

Conclusion

This paper has shown how patterns of food and beverage consumption were given ritual significance in Iron Age Veneto. Although evidence from organic remains is still too scant to propose an in-depth analysis of religious and quotidian attitudes toward eating and drinking, I suggest that an analytical emphasis on the ritual manipulation of culinary implements unearthed in graves, houses and sacred sites can augment our knowledge of ceremonial Venetic practices. Evidence from sanctuaries testifies that food consumption was one of the main cultic practices in the Veneto. Both zooarchaeological analysis of animal bones and research on culinary equipment disclose the great variety of rituals performed for the deity. Such ceremonies included libations, holocausts, banqueting and animal sacrifice. Burning of offerings and ritual breakage of ritual paraphernalia seem to have acted as means to reach the god, probably negotiating special relations between worshippers and the deity.

The ritualization of eating and drinking practices was extended to the funerary sphere with the placing of food offerings and culinary implements, sometimes ritually broken or laminated, both on the pyre and in the grave. The choice of the culinary equipment to be placed in the tomb was probably motivated by the social status of the dead, with aristocrats generally endowed with wealthier services compared to non-elite individuals. The use of culinary vessels as urns suggests a possible symbolic association of cremated individuals with food. The adoption of different funerary rituals (cremation versus inhumation) and of different kinds of vessel-urns may have implied a complex hierarchy in people's status after death, with the possibility that diverse metaphoric associations with different foods were given to individuals of different status.

A third context of the ritualization of food consumption was the placing of prestigious dining sets under the house floor. Performed at foundation rituals, such ceremonies involved the ritual breakage of vessels as well as the interment of cultic implements and culinary equipment linked to formal dining practices. The Venetic aristocracy's role in controlling and exploiting ritualized eating and drinking practices is shown by the importance given to the consumption of alcohol. The adoption of aristocratic forms of commensality is apparent, from at least the early Iron Age, by the placing of luxurious drinking equipment in elite graves such as tomb Este Ricovero 236. During the second

Iron Age (fifth to second centuries BC) local symposium practices were influenced by the importation of selected drinking vessels, revealing complex patterns of assimilation and rejection of foreign cultural impulses. The presence of Attic cups in aristocratic contexts – wealthy graves, sanctuaries and settlement quarters – shows how the control over selected forms of consumption may have created a gap between elite and non-elite social groups.

Acknowledgements

I would like to express my gratitude to Corinna Riva, Annie Gray and Naomi Sykes who first read a draft of this paper and to all the referees whose comments helped me to greatly improve my work.

References

Appadurai, A. 1981. 'Gastro-politics in Hindu South Asia', *American Ethnologist* **8**, 490–511.
Balista, C. and Ruta Serafini, A. 1998. 'La necropoli della Casa di Ricovero. Storia della ricerca', in Bianchin Citton, E., Gambacurta, G. and Ruta Serafini, A. (eds), *Presso l'Adige Ridente…Rinvenimenti Archeologici tra Este e Montagnana* (Padova), 17–28.
Bianco, L., Caimi, R., Gregagnin, R. and Manning Press, J. 1998. 'Lo scavo pluristratificato in Via Battisti 32 a Padova', *Archeologia Veneta* **20**, 3–110.
Bonomi, S. 2003. 'Ceramica attica ad Altino: nuovi dati', in Cresci Marrone, G. and Tirelli, M. (eds) *Produzioni, Merci e Commerci in Altino Preromana e Romana. Atti del Convegno. Venezia 12–14 Dicembre 2001* (Roma), 47–60.
Bray, T.L. (ed.) 2003. *The Archaeology and Politics of Food and Feasting in Early States and Empires* (New York).
Capuis, L. 2004. *I Veneti. Civiltà e Cultura di un Popolo dell'Italia Preromana* (Milano).
Capuis, L. and Chieco Bianchi A.M. 2002. 'Il Santuario sud-orientale. Reitia e i suoi devoti', in Ruta Serafini, A. (ed.) *Este. Una Città e i suoi Santuari* (Padova), 233–47.
Chapman, J. and Gaydarska, B. 2007. *Parts and Wholes. Fragmentation in Prehistoric Context* (Oxford).
Chieco Bianchi, A.M. 1987. 'Dati preliminari su alcune tombe di III secolo da Este', in Vitali, D. (ed.) *Celti ed Etruschi nell'Italia Centro-Settentrionale dal V secolo a. C. alla Romanizzazione. Atti del Colloquio Internazionale Bologna 12–14 Aprile 1985* (Imola), 191–236.
Chieco Bianchi, A.M. and Calzavara Capuis, L. 1985. *Este I. Le Necropoli di Casa di Ricovero, Casa Alfonsi e Casa Muletti Prosdocimi* (Roma).
Chieco Bianchi, A.M. and Calzavara Capuis, L. (eds.) 2006: *Este II. La Necropoli di Villa Benvenuti* (Roma).
Dammer, H. 2002. 'Il santuario sud-orientale. Le indagini recenti', in Ruta Serafini, A. (ed.) *Este. Una Città e i Suoi Santuari* (Padova), 248–53.
Dammer, H. 2002b: 'Il santuario lacustre di San Pietro Montagnon: quesiti irrisolti', in Ruta Serafini, A. (ed.) *Este. Una Città e i Suoi Santuari* (Padova), 299–303.
Dietler, M. 1990. 'Driven by drink: the role of drinking in the political economy and the case of Iron Age France', *Journal of Anthropological Archaeology* **9**, 352–406.
Dietler, M. and Hayden, B. (eds.) 2001. *Feasts: Archaeological and Ethnographic Perspectives on Food, Politics, and Power* (Washington).
Fiore, I. and Tagliacozzo, A. 2002. 'I resti ossei faunistici', in Ruta Serafini, A. (ed.) *Este. Una Città e i Suoi Santuari* (Padova), 185–97.
Frey, O.H. 1969. *Die Entstehung der Situlenkunst* (Berlin).

Goody, J. 1982. *Cooking, Class and Cuisine: A Study in Comparative Sociology* (Cambridge).

Gorini, G. and Mastrocinque, A. (eds.) 2005. *Stipi Votive delle Venezie. Altichiero, Monte Altare, Musile, Garda, Riva* (Roma).

Gregnanin, E. 2002. 'La ceramica', in Ruta Serafini, A. (ed.) *Este. Una Città e i Suoi Santuari* (Padova), 164–71.

Iaia, C. 2006. 'Servizi cerimoniali e da 'simposio' in bronzo del Primo Ferro in Italia Centro-Settentrionale', in Von Eles, P. (ed.) *La Ritualità Funeraria tra Età del Ferro e Orientalizzante in Italia. Atti del Convegno Verrucchio 26–27 Giugno 2002* (Pisa), 103–10.

Leonardi, G. 2004. 'Testimonianza greca dalla necropoli del Piovego', in Luni, M. (ed.) *Hesperia 18. I Greci in Adriatico 2* (Roma).

Lissarrague, F. 1990. *The Aesthetics of the Greek Banquet: Images of Wine and Ritual* (Princeton).

Motella De Carlo, S. 1998. 'La ricerca archeobotanica e le terre di rogo', in Bianchin Citton, E., Gambacurta, G. and Ruta Serafini, A. (eds) *Presso l'Adige Ridente…Rinvenimenti Archeologici tra Este e Montagnana* (Padova), 54–61.

Motella De Carlo, S. 2002. 'I resti botanici nel pozzo', in Ruta Serafini, A. (ed.) *Este. Una Città e i suoi Santuari* (Padova), 198–203.

Oestigaard, T. 2000. 'Sacrifices of raw, cooked and burnt humans', *Norwegian Archaeological Review* 33/1, 41–58.

Ruta Serafini, A. (ed.) 1990. *La Necropoli Paleoveneta di Via Tiepolo a Padova. Un Intervento Archeologico nella Città* (Padova).

Ruta Serafini, A. (ed.) 2002. *Este. Una Città e i Suoi Santuari* (Padova).

Ruta Serafini, A. 2003. 'Padova: Le *domus* di Via Zabarella', in Malnati, L. and Gamba M. (eds) *I Veneti dai Bei Cavalli* (Padova), 71.

Ruta Serafini, A. 2004. 'Il mondo veneto nell'Età del Ferro', in Marzatico, F. and Gleirscher, P. (eds), *Principi, Guerrieri ed Eroi fra il Danubio e il Po dalla Preistoria all'Alto Medioevo* (Trento), 277–86.

Ruta Serafini, A. and Sainati, C. 2002. 'Il "caso" Meggiaro. Problemi e prospettive', in Ruta Serafini, A. (ed.) *Este. Una Città e i suoi Santuari* (Padova), 216–23.

Schuitema, K. 2008. 'The Origins of the Archaic Greek *Symposium*: Internal Developments and Near Eastern influences', in Baker, S. Allen, M., Middle, S. And Poole, K. (eds), *Food and Drink in Archaeology 1* (Totnes).

Tirelli, M. 2002. 'Il santuario di Altino: *Altno-* e i cavalli', in Ruta Serafini, A. (ed.) *Este. Una Città e i Suoi Santuari* (Padova), 311–16.

Vitri, S. 1996. 'L'abitato e i luoghi di culto', in Malnati L., Croce da Villa, P. and Di Filippo Balestrazzi, E. (eds) *La Protostoria tra Sile e Tagliamento. Antiche Genti tra Veneto e Friuli* (Padova), 399–408.

Infant Feeding and Weaning Practices as Data for Fertility Estimates of a Roman-Period Population Sample from Kellis 2, Dakhleh Oasis, Egypt

Jennifer Sharman, University of Durham

Bioarchaeologists strive to use all available organic and inorganic evidence to study the once-living inhabitants of past cultures. Food and drink constitute an important source of evidence – and not just in terms of a possible menu of the ancient people (although, of course, diet and the items consumed are interesting research areas in their own right). By examining differences in the type or quantity of food and drink consumed between individuals using chemical analysis and other archaeological evidence, it is possible to suggest that variations in diet reflect differences in social status and/or culture (e.g. White *et al.* 1993; Ambrose *et al.* 2003; Montgomery *et al.* 2005). Age-related variation in diet may also be seen: for instance, most infants in the past would have been breastfed – if not by their own mothers then by a wet nurse – and the gradual addition of supplementary food would have led to the eventual weaning off breast milk. This process, and the associated stable carbon and nitrogen isotopic evidence contained in the bones of infants, can provide important data on the age at which infants were weaned as well as further information on fertility.

Fertility estimates gathered from archaeological populations are typically limited, due to the nature of the data. For example, fecundity, or the physiological ability to bear children, is inherently unobservable even in living populations, but can be estimated from a couple's waiting time prior to conception (Wood 1994, 88). Through censuses or interviews, demographers obtain information on age at first marriage and duration of marriage, and calculate this and other indices alongside completed parity, or number of children, for each family (Wood 1994, 38). Archaeologists rarely have information on age at marriage, duration of marriage or completed parity, particularly for prehistoric populations.

This paper presents a new model for calculating birth spacing which has used stable carbon and nitrogen isotopic weaning age data from Dupras *et al.*'s (2001) study of the Roman period Kellis 2 skeletal population from the Dakhleh Oasis, Egypt. The equations detailed here for calculating the length of birth interval have been developed from modern data for duration of lactational amenorrhea, according to intensity of breastfeeding (Smith 1985, 157). The modelled fertility parameters include estimates of birth interval, gross reproductive rate, total fertility rate, and mean completed family size, which were then correlated with modelled population growth rates for a more complete picture of the once-living population.

This work was undertaken as part of a project that modelled growth rates into the age-at-death distribution from the Kellis 2 (K2) cemetery. The question of whether the population was stationary, stable, or growing was addressed in order to make inferences and calculations of a demographic nature. Stability is a safer assumption than stationarity, and was used for K2. An in-depth discussion of paleodemographic issues is beyond the scope of this work; here it is sufficient to note that the K2 sample was deemed representative of the once-living population (Sharman 2007, 97). Archaeological and ethnographic evidence suggests that Kellis supported a growing population, particularly during the Roman period. It was reasoned that an appropriate range of annual population growth rates for K2 was from 0.5 to 1.48 per cent (Sharman 2007, 100).

The sample

The Dakhleh Oasis is located in the Western Desert of Egypt, and is approximately 2500 km^2 in area, lying around 660 kilometres south of Cairo (Dupras and Schwarcz 2001, 1199). Dakhleh always had a reliable underground water supply from the Nubian Sandstone Series, which bears a more than 30,000 year old confined aquifer (Thorweihe 1990, 601).

The town of Kellis, situated in the central part of the Dakhleh Oasis, was an important religious and commercial centre, continuously occupied from the Ptolemaic (*c.*332–27 BC) to late Roman (*c.*100–400 AD) period (Molto 2001, 98; Dupras *et al.* 2001, 204). An agrarian lifestyle predominated throughout and a wide variety of crops were grown, including barley, wheat, millet, olives, apricots and figs; nuts, sheep and goats were also part of the diet (Dupras 1999, 104). The diet changed little over time and is considered to be well balanced (Dupras 1999, 254).

The K2 cemetery is to the north-east of the archaeological town site of Kellis, and contains the remains of the occupants of the site from the later Roman period (Tocheri *et al.* 2005, 329). The hyperarid conditions of the oasis over the past several millennia have resulted in near perfect preservation of the skeletons, of which some show large amounts of preserved soft tissue. To date, over 600 K2 burials have been excavated and analysed, representing approximately 20 to 30 per cent of the site (see Figure 9.1). The K2 sample includes individuals from all age groups, including a large number of fetal remains (Tocheri *et al.* 2005, 329). Burials were single, well-preserved interments, oriented east-west, with the head in the latter direction and the body in an extended position.

Age and sex determinations were performed in the field by Dr. J.E. Molto. Fetal remains were aged using basiocciput osteometrics and ossification of long bones; for juvenile remains, dental calcification and eruption (following Ubelaker 1989, 63), and maximum length of the femoral diaphyses (following Kósa 1989, 45) were used to estimate age (Tocheri and Molto 2002, 358). K2 is a large sample, and includes the remains of many subadults, and is therefore particularly suitable for palaeodemographic

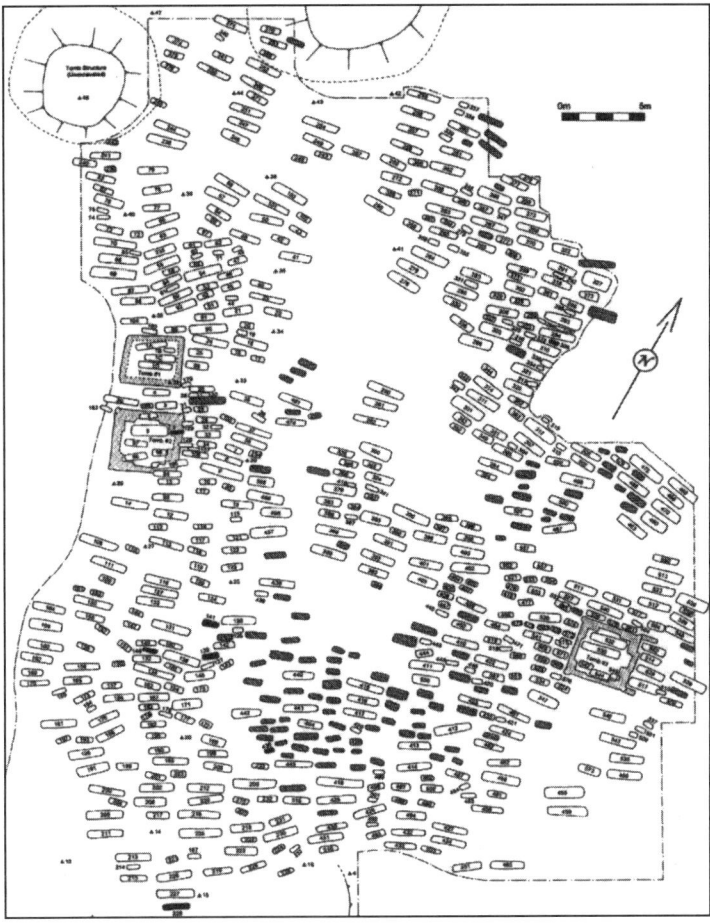

Figure 9.1. Kellis 2 cemetery: excavated portion.

research. The analysed sample consisted of 484 individuals: 226 adults comprising 93 males and 133 females ranging from 17 to 72 years of age at death; the 258 subadults included 23 perinates and 25 fetuses. Within the subadult category, the perinate to six month old group contained the highest proportion (45%) of individuals, which is as expected, given that this category is most at risk.

Dakhleh stable isotope analysis

It is widely accepted that the stable nitrogen isotope ratio measured in an animal or human reflects their trophic level of dietary protein, with ratios increasing at each step in the food chain so that a carnivore is expected to have a higher ratio than a herbivore (White *et al.* 1993, 354; Thompson *et al.* 2005, 452). This has some implications for studying breast feeding and weaning times. For instance, by feeding from another human, breast-fed infants are trophically higher, and so will have inflated nitrogen isotopic ratios compared to their mother/wet-nurse. As supplementary food is added to the infant's diet, its isotopic nitrogen ratio decreases. When weaning is complete, the nitrogen isotopic ratio of the child should be similar to that of the mother (Dupras *et al.* 2001, 205). The analysis of stable carbon isotopes can complement nitrogen analysis, as changes in the ratio of carbon isotopes indicate the introduction of supplementary food, as well as whether the supplementary food items are C_3 or C_4 based. This refers to the two different photosynthetic pathways used by plants to process CO_2. In terms of supplementary food for an infant, for example cow or goat's milk, the infant's carbon levels reflect the type of plant on which the cow or goat fed (Dupras *et al.* 2001, 206).

To investigate patterns of breastfeeding and weaning, Dupras *et al.* (2001) analysed nitrogen and carbon isotope ratios for infants from the K2 cemetery. They also considered evidence from classical sources, as Roman period documents indicate gradual weaning beginning around six months of age, introducing foods like boiled honey or a combination of honey and goat's milk, with weaning completed by three years of age (Dupras *et al.* 2001, 205). Prior to Dupras *et al.*'s study, it was uncertain whether the Roman period residents of the oasis had adopted these Roman practices. Earlier Pharaonic Egyptian documents suggest that infants were breastfed up to three years of age, with the introduction of other foods like eggs and goat, cow or sheep milk when infants were 'several months old' (Dupras *et al.* 2001, 204). The stable isotope analysis results suggest that infants were breastfed until approximately three years of age, with supplementary foods being introduced at around six months of age (Dupras *et al.* 2001, 208). Given the isotope data, it is further suggested that the likely supplementary food was goat or cow milk from animals that had fed on millet (a C_4 plant). This supports the hypothesis that weaning was gradual in the Roman period, as outlined by the great physicians of the day, Galen and Soranus (Dupras *et al.* 2001, 205). While 'lag time' – that is, the time delay between the change in diet and the resulting change in isotopic signature in the bone collagen – is unknown (Herring *et al.* 1998, 434; Richards *et al.* 2002, 209), Herring *et al.* (1998, 435) surmise that a lag time of a few months might be expected during the first year of life, given a typical infant's growth and development trajectory. However, it is noteworthy that the weaning schedule suggested by the isotopic analysis carried out by Dupras *et al.* (2001, 208) is supported by contemporary Roman documents.

Methods
The isotope data are useful for calculating fertility rates and estimating the number of children per family. Studies have shown that the correlation between breastfeeding and postpartum amenorrhea (the non-return of menses post-pregnancy) is strong (Smith 1985, 155; Khella *et al.* 2004, 317). A number of multinational studies have found that lactational amenorrhea as a method of birth control or spacing had an efficacy rate

of 98.3 to 99.1 per cent; that is, pregnancy was reported in only 0.9 to 1.7 per cent of women experiencing lactational amenorrhea up to six months after giving birth (World Health Organisation 1999, 431). Within 12 months of childbirth, during full breastfeeding, the cumulative pregnancy rates extended from 6.6 to 7.4 per cent, and up to the end of partial breastfeeding, the rates ranged from 3.7 to 5.2 per cent (World Health Organisation 1999, 431). It is noted that if lactational amenorrhea is used to control birth spacing, the intensity and frequency of breastfeeding, as well as duration, are important (Khella *et al.* 2004, 317).

In a study of 18 developing countries, Smith (1985, 157) used linear regression analysis to provide equations for computing the median birth interval in high- and moderate-fertility populations. The high-fertility populations were those defined as having a Total Fertility Rate (TFR – the number of children per woman) of five or more. The equation for estimating the birth interval for the high fertility group was given as:

[Equation 1]
median birth interval = 21 months + 0.6 x median breastfeeding duration
(r^2 = 0.71–0.77) (Smith 1985, 158).

Calculations of net reproductive rate, using the proportion of Dakhleh females surviving to the mean age of reproduction suggest that a minimum of six children would have been necessary for a growing population. The net reproductive rate (NRR), or R_0, is calculated by $R_0 = \Delta_a R$, where Δ_a is the proportion of females surviving to the mean age of reproduction, and R is the gross reproductive rate. This equation was used to estimate the birth interval for women of ancient Dakhleh, given Equation 1 and the breastfeeding duration of 36 months.

Other studies have examined the relationship between the length of postpartum amenorrhea and duration of breastfeeding. Bongaarts and Potter (1983, 25) estimated the following equation to describe this relationship:

[Equation 2]
$A = 1.753 e^{0.1396 \times B - 0.001872 \times B^2}$, ($R^2$ = 0.96)

where A is the mean or median time, in months, of postpartum amenorrhea, and B is the mean or median length in months of breastfeeding.

Bongaarts and Potter (1983, 87) provide an equation to estimate the 'index of postpartum infecundability', which is equal to one where breastfeeding and postpartum abstinence are not practised, and is equal to zero where the length of the infecund period is infinite:

[Equation 3]
$C_i = 20/18.5 + i$

where i is the mean length of time of postpartum infecundability, from lactation or postpartum abstinence.

Then, to estimate total natural marital fertility (TN) (Bongaarts and Potter 1985, 93):

[Equation 4]
TN = 15.3 x C_i

The resulting estimate of birth spacing in the ancient population was used to estimate the number of children born to each woman. In typical demographic procedures, the first postpartum menses is taken as a symptom of the return of ovulation and hence fecundity. With no access to such information here, duration of breastfeeding was used to calculate birth interval in a manner almost backwards from the usual demographic calculations. As modern Egyptian data for rural girls suggest an age at menarche of 13.89 years, and given the modern trend in industrialized countries for a decreased age at menarche (Attallah 1978, 187), it might be expected that age at menarche in Roman Egypt would be somewhat higher. The 1966 figure for Nubians in Egypt of 15.2 years at menarche provides an interesting comparison (Wood 1994, 419). As there is also a subfecund period after menarche (Chamberlain 2006, 54), an appropriate estimated starting point for age at first conception is 18 years of age. Supporting this are modern Egyptian statistics of median age at first marriage and median maternal age at first birth, of 19.7 and 21.4 respectively, and that the drop in modern total fertility has been partially attributed to a rise in age at first marriage (Aoyama 2001, 39 and 64).

This analysis assumes the uniformitarian theory in that lactational amenorrhea prevented pregnancy with a similar efficiency in ancient and modern populations. It is also assumed that the ancient population was not practicing another form of birth control or spacing, such as sexual abstinence following child birth. Further, as the breastfeeding behaviours of the mothers of Kellis cannot be observed, it must be assumed that their full breastfeeding is comparable to the full breastfeeding as practiced by women involved in the reference studies. Here, it was assumed that intensity of breastfeeding is related to the addition or nonaddition of supplementary foods to the infant's diet.

Results

For Dakhleh, where isotopic data suggest a weaning age at approximately 36 months, and using Equation 1 (Smith 1985, 158) for the median birth interval:

median birth interval = 21 *months* + 0.6 x *median breastfeeding duration*
= 42.6 months

Using 18 years as a starting point for conception, a birth interval of 42.6 months, and the last birth at 47.2 years, a woman might have up to nine children, depending on the age of menopause (see Table 9.1). As the birth interval tends to increase before the last child, following Wood (1994, 98), and menopause typically occurs around 50 years, eight or nine children may be a feasible number of births.

Parity	1	2	3	4	5	6	7	8	9
Maternal Age (years)	18.75	22.25	25.67	29.33	33.0	36.42	40.0	43.5	47.17

Table 9.1. Estimates of maternal age based on birth interval of 42.6 months.

Alternatively, using Equation 2 (Bongaarts and Potter 1983, 25) and the typical 36 months of breastfeeding, as evidenced by the stable isotope data for Dakhleh:

$$A = 1.753e^{0.1396 \times B - 0.001872 \times B^2} = 23.59 \text{ months of postpartum amenorrhea.}$$

And the index of postpartum infecundability (Equation 3; Bongaarts and Potter 1983, 87), where i is estimated by A:

$$C_i = 20/18.5 + i = 0.4752$$

From this estimate, TN can be approximated as:

$$TN = 15.3 \times C_i = 7.27056$$

Where it is assumed that all women of reproductive age were married, no contraception was used and no abortion induced, TN is equal to TFR (Bongaarts and Potter 1983, 80). While contraception may have been practiced by the women of K2, they were probably low level barrier methods or the use of substances with spermicidal properties (Riddle 1992, 67, 75). Abortion, which may have been illegal (Halioua and Ziskind 2005, 176), was probably not induced often enough to greatly affect this estimate of fertility and as such, the estimated value of TN was used as the TFR here.

Discussion

The estimates of birth interval using Smith's equation (1985, 158), and the estimate of TFR based on Bongaarts and Potter's (1983, 87) indices of conception of 7.3, provide an interesting complement to Aoyama's (2001, 38) Egyptian study, which reported a very similar TFR of approximately seven in low and low-middle income families in 1962.

Smith's equation produces a birth interval of 42.6 months, and simply counting from 18 years as the age of first conception leads to an estimate of nine children, with the last birth taking place at a maternal age of 47.2 years. However, this simple counting of the birth interval does not take into account the sub-fecund periods at the beginning and end of a female's reproductive years. Most studies of fertility note a peak in fecundity in the twenties (Chamberlain 2006, 35) and it is a well established medical fact that obstetrical problems and birth defects increase with maternal age, beginning around the mid 30s. As such, it is posited that 7.3 to eight children is probably a sound estimate of the total fertility rate at Kellis in the Roman period. However, if Dakhleh females breastfed through part or all of the next pregnancy, the birth interval would be closer to 36 months. This difference is only about seven months and extended over a lifetime of childbearing, this would probably only add one child per woman.

These figures can be used to compute mean family size, using Lutz's (1989, 83) equation:

$$x = \sum_{x=1}^{n} f(x)x \text{ where } f(x) \text{ is the proportion of females of completed parity } x$$

Using the population growth rate range of 0.5 to 1.48 per cent per annum, the mean completed family size ranges from 1.74 to 2.56 children per family. Further, given the estimated TFR of 7.3 to eight, the Gross Reproductive Rate (GRR) and Net Reproductive Rate (NRR) can be calculated. GRR is the number of daughters per woman (or TFR multiplied by the proportion of females in the population), while NRR is the same measure, but adjusted for female mortality – an important measure, as not all women would survive to the end of the reproductive years. For all growth rates, GRR extends from 3.55 to 3.90; the NRR reaches from 1.42 to 1.95 depending on the growth rate within the aforementioned range.

These estimates are based on families with completed parity. As many females did not survive until the end of the reproductive period, mean completed family size estimates were significantly lower, and ranged from 1.74 to 2.56 children per family, the lower and upper limits encompassing the range estimated for growth rates of 0.5, 1 and 1.48 per cent per year. While these estimates appear low, they are simply the mean completed family size; as suggested by the NRR, where the limiting condition is NRR = 1, which signifies a non-growing sustaining population, the growth rates and TFR range given above are all possible.

Conclusions

By using empirical evidence from skeletally-derived weaning age and ethnographic data, models of the possible fertility and mortality experiences of the ancient K2 population have been constructed. Life expectancy at birth was low but as a consequence of high fertility and high infant mortality, as women of completed parity probably gave birth to seven or eight children, with perhaps only five or six surviving past early childhood. While maternal mortality was higher than in most modern countries, the varied diet, constant water supply and uncrowded living conditions helped to sustain a growing population.

It has been demonstrated that if weaning data are available from isotopic studies, these can be used in conjunction with proposed growth rates to model fertility, including not only demographic measures such as the total fertility rate, gross reproduction rate and net reproduction rate, but also completed family size and mean completed family size. It is hoped that this method will provide a model for extracting as much fertility information as possible from skeletal populations, using all available data.

References

Ambrose, S.H., Buikstra, J. and Krueger, H.W. 2003. 'Status and gender differences in diet at Mount 72, Cahokia, revealed by isotopic analysis of bone', *Journal of Anthropological Archaeology* 22, 217–26.

Aoyama, A. 2001. *Reproductive Health in the Middle East and North Africa* (Washington).

Attallah, N.L. 1978. 'Age at menarche of schoolgirls in Egypt', *Annals of Human Biology* 5, 185–89.

Bongaarts, J. and Potter, R.G. 1983. *Fertility, Biology, and Behavior: An Analysis of the Proximate Determinants* (Toronto).

Chamberlain, A. 2006. *Demography in Archaeology* (Cambridge).

Dupras, T.L. 1999. *Dining in the Dakhleh Oasis, Egypt: Determination of Diet Using Documents and Stable Isotope Analysis* (Hamilton ON, Unpublished PhD Thesis).

Dupras, T.L. and Schwarcz, H.P. 2001. 'Strangers in a strange land: stable isotope evidence for human migration in the Dakhleh Oasis, Egypt', *Journal of Archaeological Science* 28, 1199–1208.

Dupras, T.L., Schwarcz, H.P. and Fairgrieve, S.I. 2001. 'Infant feeding and weaning practices in Roman Egypt', *American Journal of Physical Anthropology* 115, 204–12.

Halioua, B. and B. Ziskind 2005. *Medicine in the Days of the Pharaohs* (Cambridge).

Herring, D.A., Saunders, S.R. and Katzenberg, M.A. 1998. 'Investigating the weaning process in past populations', *American Journal of Physical Anthropology* 105, 425–39.

Khella, A.K., Fahim, H.I., Issa, A.H., Sokal, D.C. and Gadalla, M.A. 2004. 'Lactational amenorrhea as a method of family planning in Egypt', *Contraception* 69, 317–22.

Kósa, F. 1989. 'Age estimation from the fetal skeleton', in İşcan, M.Y. (ed.) *Age Markers in the Human Skeleton* (Springfield), 21–54.

Lutz, W. 1989. *Distributional Aspects of Human Fertility: a Global Comparative Study* (Toronto).

Molto, J.E. 2001. 'The comparative skeletal biology and paleoepidemiology of the people from Ein Tirghi and Kellis, Dakhleh, Egypt', in Marlow, C.A. and Mills, A.J. (eds.) *The Oasis Papers — Proceedings of the First International Symposium of the Dakhleh Oasis Project* (Oxford), 81–100.

Montgomery, J., Evans, J.A., Powlesland, D. and Roberts, C.A. 2005. 'Continuity or colonization in Anglo-Saxon England? Isotope evidence for mobility, subsistence practice, and status at West Heslerton', *American Journal of Physical Anthropology* 126, 123–38.

Richards, M.P., Mays, S. and Fuller, B.T. 2002. 'Stable carbon and nitrogen isotope values of bone and teeth reflect weaning age at the medieval Wharram Percy site, Yorkshire, UK', *American Journal of Physical Anthropology* 119, 205–10.

Riddle, J.M. 1992. *Contraception and abortion from the ancient world to the Renaissance* (Cambridge, MA).

Sharman, J. 2007. *Modeling fertility and demography in a Roman period population sample from Kellis 2, Dakhleh Oasis, Egypt* (Unpublished MA thesis, London ON).

Smith, D.P. 1985. 'Breastfeeding, contraception and birth intervals in developing countries. *Studies in Family Planning* 16, 154–63.

Thompson, A.H., Richards, M.P., Shortland, A. and Zakrzewski S.R. 2005. 'Isotopic palaeodiet studies of Ancient Egyptian fauna and humans', *Journal of Archaeological Science* 32, 451–63.

Thorweihe, U. 1990. 'Nubian Aquifer system', in Said, R. (ed.) *The Geology of Egypt* (Rotterdam), 601–11.

Tocheri, M.W., Dupras, T.L., Sheldrick, P. and Molto, J.E. 2005. 'Roman Period fetal skeletons from the East Cemetery (Kellis 2) of Kellis, Egypt', *International Journal of Osteoarchaeology* 15, 326–41.

Tocheri, M.W. and Molto, J.E. 2002. 'Aging fetal and juvenile skeletons from Roman Period Egypt using basiocciput osteometrics', *International Journal of Osteoarchaeology* 12, 356–63.

Ubelaker, D.H. 1989. *Human Skeletal Remains: Excavation, Analysis, Interpretation* (Washington).

White, C.D., Healy, P.F. and Schwarcz, H.P. 1993. 'Intensive agriculture, social status and Maya diet at Pacbitun, Belize', *Journal of Anthropological Research* 49, 347–75.

Wood, J.W. 1994. *Dynamics of Human Reproduction: Biology, Biometry and Demography* (New York).

World Health Organization Task Force on Methods for the Natural Regulation of Fertility. 1999. 'The World Health Organization multinational study of breast-feeding and lactational amenorrhea. III. Pregnancy during breast-feeding', *Fertility and Sterility* 72, 431–40.

Stable Isotope Analysis of DISH and Diet

Rosa Spencer,
University of Durham

Diffuse idiopathic skeletal hyperostosis (DISH) is a disorder characterised by hyperostosis and ankylosis of the spinal column on the antero-lateral side, and also ossification of extra-spinal entheses and ligaments (Pappone *et al.* 1996; Rogers and Waldron 2001). The spinal bone fusion is often described as a 'flowing' ossification that resembles dripping candle-wax and is usually located on the right-hand side of the thoracic vertebrae (the presence of the aorta preventing ossification on the opposite side) and on either the right or left-hand side of the lumbar vertebrae (Mader 2002; Reale *et al.* 1999; Sarzi-Puttini and Atzeni 2004).

Today DISH occurs in men and women over 40 years of age with a ratio of 2:1, and its frequency and severity increase with age and body weight (Camimisa *et al.* 1998; el Miedany *et al.* 2000; Sarzi-Puttini and Atzeni 2004). In archaeological populations, the prevalence rates indicate that DISH is a common occurrence in medieval monastic communities with reported rates of DISH being 8.6 per cent at Merton Priory, Surrey (Waldron 1985, 1763); 13.4 per cent amongst those over 40 years of age at Blackfriars Friary, Ipswich (Mays 1991, 122); 9.1 per cent at Wells Cathedral (Rogers and Waldron 2001, 360), and 19 per cent at the Basilica of Saint Servaas, Maastricht (Janssen and Maat 1999). Waldron (1985) and Rogers and Waldron (2001) believe that these high prevalence rates may be attributable to a 'high-status' lifestyle and, in particular, to a high calorie, high animal protein diet. These suggested links with monasticism have recently been questioned by Mays (2006) and Oxenham *et al.* (2006) but have not yet been properly tested.

Other theories regarding the aetiology of DISH exist (for example, links with trauma, environment, physiology, and genetics – see Childs 2004, Crubezy 1996, Havelka *et al.* 2001, Havelka *et al.* 2002, Gorman *et al.* 2006, Greenfield and Goldberg 1997, Macones *et al.* 1989, Pappone *et al.* 1996, Rogers *et al.* 1997), but the idea that DISH results from over-eating and a diet rich in animal protein has become established in the osteoarchaeological literature. Consequently, the presence of DISH is frequently used as an indicator of high status. However, my research is testing the theory that DISH is linked to high animal protein diet using carbon and nitrogen stable isotope analysis to see if differences in diet exist between those individuals with DISH and those without.

Stable Isotope Analysis of DISH and Diet

Stable isotope analysis and DISH

Stable isotope analysis is used to reconstruct diet at the level of the individual, so differences in carbon and nitrogen isotope values are to be expected within the populations under study. The use of stable isotopes in diet reconstruction is based on the principle 'you are what you eat'. Isotopic analysis of consumer bone collagen provides a dietary signature, which represents an average of the foods consumed over the last 10–30 years before death (Hedges *et al.* 2007). In the temperate environment of late medieval Britain, the foods derived primarily from a C_3 ecosystem. Therefore any differences in the carbon isotope signature ($\delta^{13}C$) are likely to reflect variations in the consumption of terrestrial and marine protein (Chisholm *et al.* 1982; DeNiro and Epstein 1978; Müldner and Richards 2005).

The nitrogen isotope ratio value ($\delta^{15}N$) increases with every step in the food chain, known as the "trophic level effect" (Ambrose *et al.* 2003; Fuller *et al.* 2003). Therefore, $\delta^{15}N$ values can be used to identify a diet derived mainly from plant or animal protein. The consumption of aquatic foods can also be identified because they exhibit significantly higher $\delta^{15}N$ values compared to terrestrial animals, most likely due to the longer food chains in aquatic environments that result in the accumulation of more trophic levels (Privat *et al.* 2002). The use of both isotope systems could help to potentially identify the consumption of omnivore and freshwater protein in the diet (Müldner and Richards 2005).

There are, of course, many factors to consider when analysing diet but, in very general terms, an omnivorous diet high in animal protein can be distinguished from an omnivorous diet containing less animal protein. In terms of analysing DISH, this means that any correlations between those individuals with DISH and those individuals with diets high in animal protein will be identified and it should be possible to determine if links exist between diet and DISH. Stable isotope analysis has rarely been utilised as a tool to study disease; this research provides a unique opportunity to expand the current applications of carbon and nitrogen stable isotope analysis and also to enhance the understanding of a disease about which very little is known. The focus of this paper is to discuss the $\delta^{15}N$ values for those individuals with and without DISH and to determine whether this provides evidence for a relationship between DISH and diet.

Materials and methods

Small pieces of bone (1–2 g) from ribs were sampled from skeletal material from late medieval (twelfth to sixteenth century) sites in Britain. Samples were taken from nine sites – four monastic and five non-monastic. The monastic sites, which include of a number of different monastic orders, were St. James Abbey in Northampton (Augustinian), Blackfriars Friary in Gloucester (Dominican), Merton Priory in Surrey (Augustinian), and the Abbey of St. Mary Graces in London (Cistercian). The non-monastic sites were Fishergate House in York, Hereford Cathedral in Hereford, the leprosy Hospital of St. James and St. Mary Magdalene in Chichester, the Royal Mint Black Death cemetery in

London, and Blackfriars Friary in Ipswich (Dominican). Whilst the last site is monastic, the skeletal material, according to Mays (1991), represents the lay benefactors rather than monks and is therefore grouped with the non-monastic samples. As DISH is a condition that affects older individuals, only adults over 40 years of age were sampled. A minimum of three contiguously fused (or fused and broken post-mortem) vertebrae were used for diagnosis of DISH.

In total, 46 bone samples were analysed– 40 males and six females; 23 with DISH and 23 without; 25 monastic and 21 non-monastic (see Table 1). Collagen was extracted from each of these bone samples using methods described in Richards and Hedges (1999) with an added filtration step (Brown *et al.* 1988). Essentially, the bone was demineralised, gelatinised, purified by ultrafiltration, and then freeze-dried to obtain the resulting collagen. The collagen was weighed out into tin capsules in 0.25–0.35 mg batches and then analysed via continuous-flow isotope ratio mass spectrometry in the Alaska Stable Isotope Facility at the University of Alaska Fairbanks' Water & Environmental Research Center. Samples were run in duplicate and the $\delta^{13}C$ and $\delta^{15}N$ values averaged to produce a single reading for each sample. Any samples that fell outside the acceptable range for C/N ratios of 2.4 –3.6, as recommended by Ambrose (1990) and DeNiro (1985), were discarded.

The resulting $\delta^{13}C$ and $\delta^{15}N$ values were plotted on a series of scatterplots and the values were compared between different groups – for example, male and females, monastic and non-monastic, those with DISH and those without – using Mann-Whitney tests to assess statistical significant differences at the 5 per cent level.

Results

The data sets for the various groupings of male versus female and monastic versus non-monastic yielded no significant differences at the 5 per cent level for both $\delta^{13}C$ and $\delta^{15}N$ values. For the purposes of this paper, only the results for the groups with and without DISH will be considered; these are summarised in Table 10.1 together with data for the other groups (for raw data see Spencer in prep.). The results of the statistical analysis indicate that there is a significant difference (at the 5 per cent level) in $\delta^{15}N$ values between those skeletons with DISH and those without and also between monastic skeletons with and without DISH. However, there is no significant difference in $\delta^{15}N$ values between males with and without the disease.

Discussion

The absence of any significant differences in $\delta^{15}N$ values for males with and without DISH is important considering that the majority of the dataset (40 of 46 samples) are males. The significant differences found amongst all skeletons with and without DISH could be due to sample size or the small group of six female skeletons skewing the data when examining all skeletons together; but the significant differences amongst monastic skeletons with and without DISH is difficult to explain, given that they are all males.

Stable Isotope Analysis of DISH and Diet

Data	Mean δ^{13}C	Mean δ^{15}N	Significant Difference in δ^{13}C	Significant Difference in δ^{15}N
Skeletons with and without DISH	-19.9‰ +/-0.56‰ (DISH n=23) -20.1‰ +/- 0.64‰ (non-DISH n=23)	13.4‰ +/- 0.79‰ (DISH n=23) 12.7‰ +/- 1.1‰ (non-DISH n=23)	0.258	**0.012**
Monastic skeletons with and without DISH	-19.9‰ +/- 0.71‰ (DISH n=14) -20.4‰ +/- 1.2‰ (non-DISH n=11)	13.4‰ +/- 0.89‰ (DISH n=14) 12.5‰ +/- 1.2‰ (non-DISH n=11)	0.134	**0.003**
Male skeletons with and without DISH	-19.9‰ +/- 0.58‰ (DISH n=21) -20.1‰ +/- 1.1‰ (non-DISH n=19)	13.4‰ +/- 0.82‰ (DISH n=21) 12.9‰ +/- 1.1‰ (non-DISH n=19)	0.436	0.074
Monastic skeletons versus non-monastic skeletons	-20.4‰ +/- 0.62‰ (monastic n=25) -20.0‰ +/- 0.59‰ (non-monastic n=21)	13.2‰ +/- 0.96‰ (monastic n=25) 12.6‰ +/- 1.1‰ (non-monastic n=21)	0.385	0.474
Male skeletons versus female skeletons	-19.9‰ +/-0.6‰ (males n=40) -20.0‰ +/- 0.5‰ (females n=6)	13.2‰ +/- 0.9‰ (males n=40) 12.6‰ +/- 1.3‰ (females n=6)	0.379	0.453

Table 10.1. Summary of results of Mann-Whitney tests. Results in bold are significant at the 5 per cent level. For raw data see Spencer (in prep.).

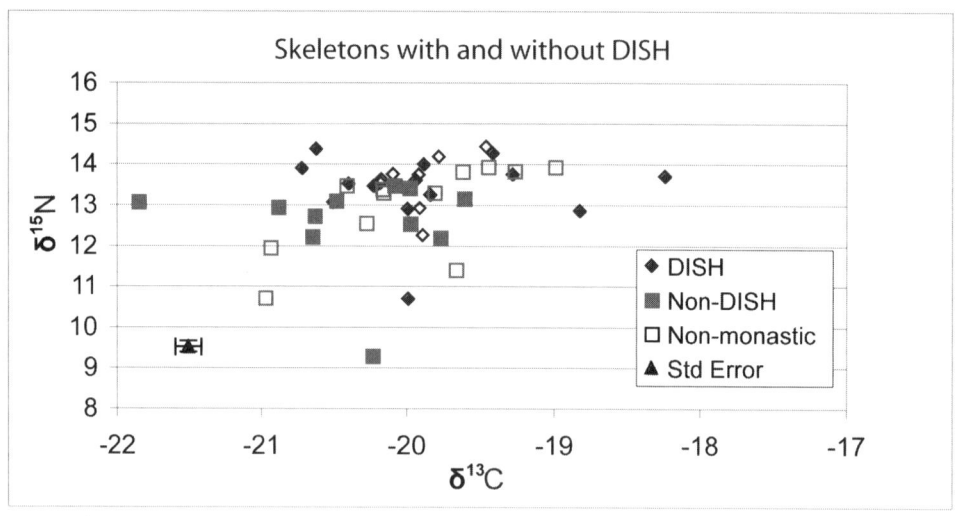

Figure 10.1 Skeletons with and without DISH. Non-monastic skeletons are shown in open symbols, monastic skeletons are shown as solid symbols.

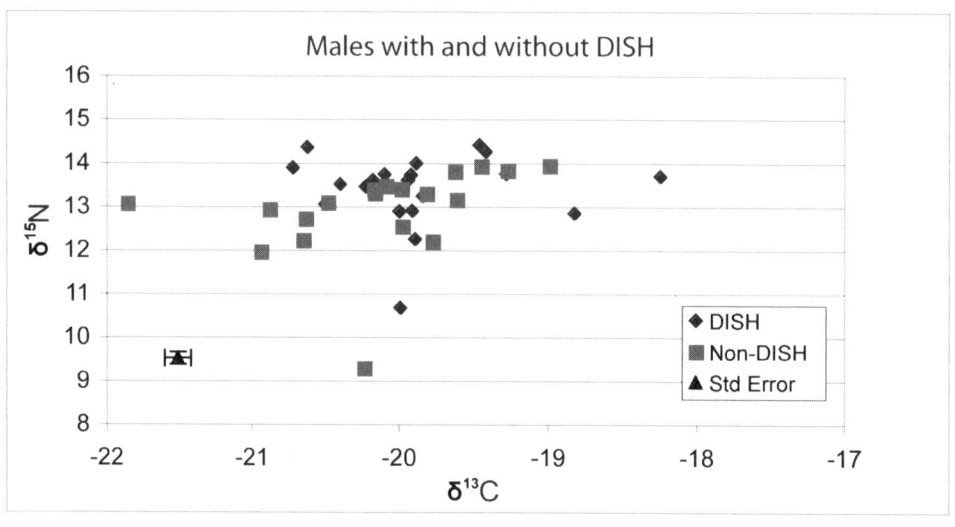

Figure 10.2. Males with and without DISH.

Stable Isotope Analysis of DISH and Diet

The scatterplots of the data for these groups show visual differences between those with DISH and those without in all three comparisons – the individuals with DISH appear to have more elevated $\delta^{15}N$ values than those without. If the significant differences in $\delta^{15}N$ values are due to DISH then it would be expected that the males with and without DISH would also show significant differences in $\delta^{15}N$, but they do not. This implies some other influence(s), possibly due to the small group of female samples or monasticism. Unfortunately, the female sample size is too small to assess any sex-related dietary differences and the comparison of monastic and non-monastic groups suggests that there are no isotopic differences between these two groups.

Since fasting regulations were expected to be upheld by all members of society, not just the religious, an absence of differences between the monastic and non-monastic groups is not entirely surprising. However, one might expect the monastic orders to be more dedicated in their upholding of the monastic rule and therefore produce some isotopic differences. The Rules of St Benedict and St Augustine, to which monastic communities were expected to adhere, prohibited meat from being eaten as it was thought to invoke carnal desire and distract the mind from prayer (Tobin 1995, 136). Fish was allowed to be substituted though, and game was consumed on certain occasions (Gasquet 1922, 52; Lawrence 1990, 31, 79). It is unclear from the documentary evidence how closely these rules were followed, with accounts of monastic communities sending out dogs to hunt pigs and thus 'transform' them into game, tales of extravagant feasts, or stories of monks making claims that they were ill in order to stay in the infirmary where meat was allowed to be eaten to fortify themselves after a period of illness (Gasquet 1922, 58–59; Waldron 1985; Burton 2000, 167). Most of these accounts come from the wealthier monastic houses of the Benedictines, the documentary evidence for many of the other orders indicating that they were more austere, strictly observing the rules. Unfortunately, although differences in meat consumption and the high amounts of fish that were eaten should have resulted in differences in $\delta^{15}N$ values, they do not, nor can they account for the statistically-significant differences seen amongst DISH/non-DISH and monastic DISH/non-DISH samples in this study.

There are other, non-dietary, influences that might be possible factors for the significant differences observed in the $\delta^{15}N$ values. These include poor quality collagen, disease, dehydration, the physiological effects of fasting, and demography.

Poor quality collagen

Poor collagen yields of less than 5 per cent of the sample weight can elevate $\delta^{13}C$ and $\delta^{15}N$ values, due to the presence of contaminants from the burial environment (White and Schwarcz 1994). Any samples used in this research study which had poor yields *and* poor C/N ratios were discarded. Fewer than 10 samples with poor yields are included in the study but even these have greater than 3.5 per cent yields. Some authors maintain that when using ultrafiltration, any yield greater than 0.1 per cent is considered valid as this step greatly reduces the resulting amount of collagen (Fischer *et al.* 2007). If collagen yields are affecting the results it would be expected that both $\delta^{13}C$ and $\delta^{15}N$ would be affected. However, only the $\delta^{15}N$ values are affected so it is not likely that poor collagen yield is a factor in this case.

Disease

Katzenberg and Lovell's (1999) paper demonstrated that pathological bone produces higher $\delta^{15}N$ values than non-pathological bone. In this study of DISH, although primarily a study of disease, none of the areas of bone sampled were affected by DISH and there were no observable active or healed lesions on the ribs. One possible exception where disease may have affected the bone is the samples from the Royal Mint Black Death Cemetery. These individuals are likely to have died of plague, but it is unlikely that an infection with such a fast disease course could affect the isotope results of a slow metabolic tissue such as bone collagen. It is doubtful that disease is influencing the difference in $\delta^{15}N$ values observed in this research. However, there could be underlying disease processes which have not yet manifested themselves as skeletal changes but still influence the $\delta^{15}N$ values.

Dehydration

Animal studies have shown that dehydration can elevate $\delta^{15}N$ values in the body due to preferential excretion of ^{14}N through urea (Ambrose 1991). It has been hypothesised that water-stress can also elevate $\delta^{15}N$ values in humans (White and Armelagos 1997). Since monastic communities had very proscribed daily routines with specific periods set aside for eating and drinking (Lawrence 1990, 115–118; Burton 2000, 160–161), it is possible that dehydration may have influenced the statistically-significant differences seen in the $\delta^{15}N$ values. However, given that there are no statistically significant differences between monastic and non-monastic groups, it is unlikely.

Fasting

Long periods of fasting have also been known to increase ^{15}N levels as a result of recycling nitrogen from proteins broken down in the body (Macko *et al.* 1999). Assuming that the strict monastic regimes were followed, monastic communities fasted several times throughout the year, especially during Easter, with some orders consuming only bread and water (Hinnebusch 1965, 359). In addition, they had a restricted food intake for most of the winter when they were only allowed a single daily meal (Knowles 1948, 18). These periods of fasting could lead to increased ^{15}N levels but, given that there are no differences in $\delta^{15}N$ values between monastic and non-monastic groups, it seems an unlikely explanation for the statistically significant differences seen in this study.

Demography

Monastic populations are populations of males, mostly older adult males. As DISH is a condition which affects older adult males, it is not surprising that it has a high prevalence amongst monastic groups. The association with late medieval monastic groups in particular is most likely a sample bias as the number of skeletons representing the late medieval period is more than double that of any other period (see Roberts and Cox 2008:23). As all the samples chosen in this study were taken from older adults, thereby controlling for age, it is unlikely that any differences in $\delta^{15}N$ values between DISH and non-DISH groups are reflecting differences in old versus young individuals.

Conclusion

In conclusion, the significant differences in $\delta^{15}N$ values observed between the different groupings could be influenced by factors other than diet. Although dehydration and fasting are unlikely explanations, disease could certainly be a factor. Given the osteological paradox, that skeletons that do not exhibit any lesions may have been diseased individuals that died before any indicators could manifest skeletally (Wood *et al.* 1992), there is a possibility that disease could be influencing the $\delta^{15}N$ values seen and that the differences could be attributed to physiological rather than dietary processes. This could also explain why the scatterplots show DISH samples as plotting higher in $\delta^{15}N$ than non-DISH samples, even when this is not supported by the statistics. Alternatively, if we assume that the differences in $\delta^{15}N$ values reflect dietary differences, then the fact that the pattern of high $\delta^{15}N$ values for DISH samples occurs in non-monastic as well as monastic samples suggests that DISH is not a monastic phenomenon, as has been inferred by other authors such as Mays (2006) and Oxenham *et al.* (2006). The suggestion that DISH has a high prevalence amongst monastic communities is more likely to be a reflection of the demography of monastic cemeteries – that they contain high proportions of older males, rather than a reflection of their dietary practices.

Ultimately, more data and balanced sample sizes are needed in order to further explore whether differences exist between monastic and non-monastic groups, as well as between males and females, and different monastic orders. Unfortunately, the question about whether DISH is linked to monastic life and a diet rich in animal protein cannot be definitively answered with this data, but it is clear that the link between DISH and a high animal protein diet, if it indeed exists, is not strong enough to be observed in all groups of skeletons with DISH.

Acknowledgments

This research has been funded by NERC (Natural Environment Research Council) NER/S/A/2004/12245.

References

Ambrose, S.H. 1990. 'Preparation and characterization of bone and tooth collagen for isotopic analysis', *Journal of Archaeological Science* 17, 431–51.

Ambrose, S.H. 1991. 'Effect of diet, climate and physiology on nitrogen isotope abundances in terrestrial foodwebs', *Journal of Archaeological Science* 18, 293–318.

Ambrose, S.H, Buikstra, J. and Krueger, H. 2003. 'Status and gender difference in diet at Mound 72, Cahokia, revealed by isotopic analysis of bone', *Journal of Anthropological Archaeology* 22, 217–26.

Brown, T.A., Nelson, D., Vogel, J.S. and Southon, J. 1988. 'Improved collagen extraction by modified longin method'. *Radiocarbon* 30, 171–7.

Burton, J. 2000. *Monastic and Religious Orders in Britain, 1000–1300* (Cambridge).

Camimisa, M., De Serio, A. and Guglielmi, G. 1998. 'Diffuse idiopathic skeletal hyperostosis', *European Journal of Radiology* 27, S7–S11.

Childs, S. G. 2004: Diffuse idiopathic skeletal hyperostosis. *Orthopaedic Nursing* 23, 375–382.

Chisholm, B., Nelson, D. and Schwarcz, H. 1982. 'Stable–carbon isotope ratios as a measure of marine versus terrestrial protein in ancient diets', *Science* 216, 1131–2.

Crubezy, E. 1996. 'Etiopathogenesis of skeletal hyperostosis: a study of a European population that lived 7700 years ago', *Revue du Rhumatisme* 63, 481–4.

DeNiro, M. 1985. 'Postmortem preservation and alteration of *in vivo* bone collagen isotope ratios in relation to palaeodietary reconstruction', *Nature* 317, 806–9.

DeNiro, M. and Epstein, S. 1978. 'Influence of diet on the distribution of carbon isotopes in animals', *Geochimica et Cosmochimica Acta* 42, 495–506.

el Miedany, Y., Wassif, G. and Baddini, M.E.L. 2000. 'Is DISH of vascular etiology?', *Clinical and Experimental Rheumatology* 18, 193–200.

Fischer, A., Olsen, J., Richards, M., Heinemeier, J., Sveinbjörnsdóttir, Á. and Bennike, P. 2007. 'Coast-inland mobility and diet in the Danish Mesolithic and Neolithic: evidence from stable isotope values of humans and dogs', *Journal of Archaeological Science* 34, 2125–50.

Fuller, B., Richards, M. and Mays, S. 2003. 'Stable carbon and nitrogen isotope variations in tooth dentine serial sections from Wharram Percy', *Journal of Archaeological Science* 30, 1673–84.

Gasquet, C.A. 1922. *Monastic Life in the Middle Ages: With a Note on Great Britain and the Holy See 1792–1806* (London).

Gorman, C., Jawad, A. and Chikanza, I. 2006. 'A family with diffuse idiopathic skeletal hyperostosis', *Annals of the Rheumatic Diseases* 64, 1794–5.

Greenfield, E. and Goldberg, VM. 1997. 'Genetic determination of bone density', *The Lancet* 350, 1263–4.

Havelka, S., Vesela, M., Pavelkova, A. and Ruzickova, S. 2001. 'Are DISH and OPLL genetically related?', *Annals of the Rheumatic Diseases* 60, 902–3.

Havelka, S., Uitterlinden, A.G., Fang, Y., Arp, P.P., Pavelkova, A., Vesela, M., Halman, L., Forejtova, S., Ruzickova, S. and Pavelka, K. 2002. 'Collagen type I(alpha 1) and vitamin D receptor polymorphisms in diffuse idiopathic skeletal hyperostosis', *Clinical Rheumatology* 21, 347–8.

Hedges, R.E, Clement, J.G., Thomas, C.D. and O'Connell, T.C. 2007. 'Collagen turnover in the adult femoral mid-shaft: modeled from anthropogenic radiocarbon tracer measurements', *American Journal of Physical Anthropology* 133, 808–16

Hinnebusch, W. 1965. *The History of the Dominican Order: Origin and Growth to 1500* (New York).

Janssen, H. and Maat, G.J.R. 1999. 'Canons buried in the stiftskapel of the Saint Servaas Basilica at Maastricht', *Barge's. Anthropologica* 5, 1–43.

Katzenberg, M.A. and Lovell, N. 1999. 'Stable isotope variation in pathological bone', *International Journal of Osteoarchaeology* 9, 316–24.

Knowles, D. 1948. *The Religious Orders in England* (Cambridge).
Labarge, M.W. 2003. *Mistress, Maids and Men: Baronial Life in the Thirteenth Century* (London).
Lawrence, C. 1990. *Medieval Monasticism: Forms of Religious Life in Western Europe in the Middle Ages* (London).
Macko, S.A., Engel, M.H., Andrusevich, V., Lubec, G., O'Connell, T. and Hedges, R. 1999. 'Documenting the diet in ancient human populations through stable isotope analysis of hair', *Philosophical Transactions of the Royal Society of London B* 354, 65–76.
Macones Jr., A.J., Fisher, M.S. and Locke, J.L. 1989. 'Stress-related rib and vertebral changes', *Radiology* 170, 117–9.
Mader, R. 2002. 'Clinical manifestations of diffuse idiopathic skeletal hyperostosis of the cervical spine', *Seminars in Arthritis & Rheumatism* 32, 130–5.
Mays, S. 1991. *Part II: Appendix for the Medieval Burials for the Blackfriars Friary, School Street, Ipswich, Suffolk (Excavated 1983–85)*. (Ancient Monuments Laboratory report 16/91 (Part 1), London).
Mays, S. 2006. 'The osteology of monasticism in medieval England', in Gowland, R. and Knusel, C. (eds.) *Social Archaeology of Funerary Remains* (Oxford), 179–89.
Müldner, G. and Richards, M. 2005. 'Fast or feast: reconstructing diet in later medieval England by stable isotope analysis', *Journal of Archaeological Science* 32, 39–48.
Oxenham, M.F., Matsumura, H. and Nishimoto, T. 2006. 'Diffuse idiopathic skeletal hyperostosis in Late Jomon Hokkaido, Japan', *International Journal of Osteoarchaeology* 16, 34–46.
Pappone, N., Di Girolamo, C., Del Puente, A., Scarpa, R. and Oriente, P. 1996. 'Diffuse idiopathic skeletal hyperostosis (DISH): a retrospective analysis', *Clinical Rheumatology* 15, 121–4.
Privat, K., O'Connell, T. and Richards, M. 2002. 'Stable isotope analysis of human and faunal remains from the Anglo-Saxon cemetery at Berinsfield, Oxfordshire: dietary and social implications', *Journal of Archaeological Science* 29, 779–90.
Reale, B., Marchi, D. and Borgognini Tarli, S.M. 1999. 'A case of diffuse idiopathic skeletal hyperostosis (DISH) from a medieval necropolis in Southern Italy', *International Journal of Osteoarchaeology* 9, 369–73.
Richards, M. and Hedges, R. 1999. 'Stable isotope evidence for similarities in the types of marine foods used by Late Mesolithic humans at sites along the Atlantic coast of Europe', *Journal of Archaeological Science* 26, 717–22.
Roberts, C. A. and M. Cox. 2003. *Health and Disease in Britain: From Prehistory to the Present Day* (Stroud).
Rogers, J., Shepstone, L. and Dieppe, P. 1997. 'Bone formers: osteophyte and enthesophyte formation are positively associated', *Annals of the Rheumatic Diseases* 56, 85–90.
Rogers, J. and Waldron, T. 2001. 'DISH and the monastic way of life', *International Journal of Osteoarchaeology* 11, 357–65.
Sarzi-Puttini, P. and Atzeni, F. 2004. 'New developments in our understanding of DISH (diffuse idiopathic skeletal hyperostosis)', *Current Opinion in Rheumatology* 16, 287–92.
Spencer, R.K. In prep. *Testing Hypotheses about the Aetiology of DISH using Stable Isotope Analysis and Other Techniques* (Durham, Unpublished PhD Thesis)
Tobin, S. 1995. *The Cistercians: Monks and Monasteries of Europe* (London).
Waldron, T. 1985. 'DISH at Merton Priory: evidence for a "new" occupational disease?', *British Medical Journal* 291, 1762–3.
White, C.D. and Armelagos, G.J. 1997. 'Osteopenia and stable isotope ratios in bone collagen of Nubian female mummies', *American Journal of Physical Anthropology* 103, 185–99.
White, C.D. and Schwarcz, H. 1994. 'Temporal trends in stable isotopes for Nubian mummy tissues', *American Journal of Physical Anthropology* 93, 165–87.
Wood, J.W., Milner, G.R., Harpending, H.C. and Weiss, K.M. 1992. 'The osteological paradox: problems of inferring prehistoric health from skeletal samples', *Current Anthropology* 33, 343–70.

Agricultural Crop Choices and Social Change in the Yellow River Valley, North Central China during the Late Neolithic and Early Bronze Age

Alison Weisskopf,
University College London

The Mid/Late Neolithic and Early Bronze Age in north central China saw great socio-economic change, from egalitarian villages during the Yangshao period (4900–3000 BC) to more hierarchical social organization during the Longshan (3000–1850 BC) to the rise of complex societies and the emergence of the first city state at Erlitou in the Early Bronze Age Erlitou Period (1850–1100 BC) (Liu 2004, 4; Ma 2005, 3). This paper will examine whether social developments are charted by changes in agricultural crop choices.

Archaeobotanical data from phytolith (silica bodies formed in the epidermis of plants) samples collected from four archaeological sites: Xipo, Erlitou, Huizui and Baligang, in Henan, north central China (Figure 11.1), have been used to examine changes in the crop repertoire, from broomcorn millet (*Panicum miliaceum*) to foxtail millet (*Setaria italica*) to rice (*Oryza sativa*).

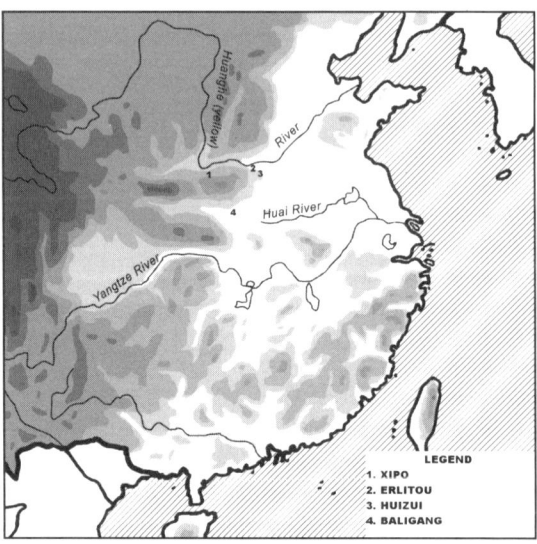

Figure 11.1. Map of China showing site distribution.

Agricultural Crop Choices and Social Change

Cultural Period and Site	Archaeological Period	Cultural Signatures	Forms of Food Production	Climate North Central China
Erlitou 1850 - 1100 BC Erlitou, Huizui West	BRONZE AGE	Differentiation between and within sites, emergence of first urban centre at Erlitou, 4 tiered hierarchy.	Large non-food producing population, dependence on surplus production of large hinterland.	Dry. Climatic fluctuations around 2000 BC.
Late Longshan 2500 –1850 BC Huizui East, Baligang	Terminal NEOLITHIC	Differentiation between sites based on household size and hierarchical complexity. Increase in site numbers.	Short fallow systems. Agricultural intensification.	Abrupt cooling period, cooler and drier.
Early Longshan 3000 – 2500 BC Huizui East, Baligan	Late NEOLITHIC	Evidence of specialization, 2 and 3 tiered hierarchies, decentralized or competing settlement system. Drop in settlement numbers.	Agricultural intensification. Expansion of anthropogenic habitats.	Mild and humid.
Late Yangshao 3500 – 3000 BC Baligang, Huizui East	Middle NEOLITHIC	Settlement hierarchy, walled settlements.	Greater intensities of crop production and land disturbance.	Mid Holocene climatic optimum.
Mid Yangshao 4000 – 3500 BC Xipo	Middle NEOLITHIC	Range of settlement types, emergence of settlement hierarchy and social differentiation.	Short fallow, permanent fields, hoe farming.	Warmer & more humid than present.
Early Yangshao 4900 – 4000 BC	Middle NEOLITHIC	Early farmer kin/work group size, small unstratified villages.	Short fallow or swidden systems. Harvesting knives increase, sickles decrease.	Mid Holocene climatic optimum.

Table 11.1. Chronology and climate in Henan, China (sources: An et al. 2000, 2006; Lee 2004, 186; Lee et al. 2007, 1091; Liu 1996, 268-269; Liu and Chen 2003, 29; Liu et al. 2004, 75, 85-86; Lu 2002, 12; Ma 2005, 100-101; Underhill 1997, 126; Xiao et al. 2004).

Agricultural Crop Choices and Social Change

Sites

Xipo is a 40-hectare mid-Yangshao single-component site in the Sha River valley, 460–472 metres above sea level (Ma 2005, 16). Erlitou is sited 10–70 metres above the riverbeds in the Yilou River Valley, a large fertile alluvial basin on a loess tableland (Lee 2004, 173; Liu *et al.* 2004, 77), with the Yellow River and Mangling Hills to the north and mountain ranges on all other sides. The Erlitou samples were collected from a palace area.

Fifteen kilometres south-east of Erlitou and five kilometres north of the Songshan Mountains, Huizui is a 40 hectare, multi-component site situated around 20 metres above the Liujian River on a Late Pleistocene terrace of alluvial silts, (Ford 2004, 71; Liu and Chen 2003, 66; Liu *et al.* 2004; Rosen 2007, 42). Liu *et al.* (2004, 91) suggest Huizui was a regional centre during the Neolithic Yangshao and Longshan cultures developing into a secondary regional centre of the Erlitou Culture.

Lying between the millet farming areas of the north and rice cultivation regions of southern China, the late Neolithic site of Baligang is situated in the northern catchment of the Yangtze River in the northern margins of the Yangtze subtropical zone inside Nanyang Basin, approximately 100–140 metres above sea level (Jiang and Zhang 1998, 66).

Chronology and climate

These sites and samples cover a temporal range from the Yangshao (4900–3000 BC) to the Longshan (3000–1850 BC) to the Erlitou (1850–1100 BC) periods, Mid Neolithic to Late Neolithic to Early Bronze Age. Palaeoecological studies have demonstrated considerable climatic and environmental change between the Yangshao and Erlitou periods (An *et al.* 2004; An *et al.* 2006; Dykoski *et al.* 2005; Herzschuh *et al.* 2004; Maher and Hu 2006; Rosen 2007; Wu and Liu 2004). The climate gradually warmed and ameliorated to a peak during the Mid-Holocene Climatic Optimum, followed by an abrupt cooling and drying and a subsequent unstable period of climatic fluctuations (Table 11.1).

There is evidence for floodplain activity and landscape alteration on the Loess Plateau (Feng *et al.* 2004; Feng *et al.* 2006). Rosen's (2007) geoarchaeological study of the Liujian River floodplain at Huizui demonstrates a marked change from a stable landscape in the early Neolithic to a strong erosive stream flow at the beginning of the Late Yangshao period, closely followed by a waterlogged marshy landscape inter cut by small streams probably brought about by the increasing precipitation during the Mid-Holocene Climatic Optimum. The valleys filled with fertile clays and silts brought in by annual flooding from amplified stream activity providing more land for cultivation, in particular the expansion of rice agriculture. This came to an abrupt end around 2400–2000 cal. BC when climatic conditions became markedly cooler and drier. At Huizui the stream cut through the sediments deposited during the Yangshao and Longshan periods drastically reducing the land available for irrigation and paddy farming (Feng *et al.* 2004; Rosen 2007, 46; Shi *et al.* 1993).

Agricultural Crop Choices and Social Change

Broad temporal changes in the agricultural economy might be determined by crop changes, which may include the introduction of new crop plants, and variation in relative proportions of millets (foxtail versus broomcorn) versus rice over the different cultural periods. Charred seed evidence suggests millets, in particular foxtail and to a lesser extent broomcorn, were the primary crop during the Yangshao in north-central China (Lee and Bestel 2007, 51). According to archaeobotanical evidence for Mid Neolithic crop distribution broomcorn was more common in the western arid interior, while foxtail was predominant in wetter eastern areas (Chang 1986; Lee *et al.* 2007, 1088). Broomcorn may be a useful insurance against drought as it is tolerant of drier conditions than foxtail or rice (Underhill 1997, 117).

The introduction of new crop plants, such as rice, which needs a constant water supply, may provide insight to variation in local environment, both natural and human induced. The introduction of rice might also affect labour and social organization, as cultivation can be labour intensive, and construction of paddies would require organized labour mobilization both to build and maintain (Netting 1993, 41). Temporal variation in the presence or absence of rice may demonstrate when rice cultivation came to the fore or declined.

Methods

This is a preliminary dataset from 40 phytolith assemblages collected from ash middens, house floors and laminated pit layers from the four sites. The majority are from homogenous ash pit fills, which were formed over time and represent several dumping episodes from secondary and tertiary deposits. They are likely to be time-averaged longer duration fills and represent the routine background noise to life.

The phytoliths were identified using a reference collection created from modern plant material collected from China and housed at the Herbarium at the Institute of Archaeology at UCL.

An advantage of using phytolith data is the possibility of distinguishing between plant parts such as seed husk and leaf/stem. This affords the opportunity of identifying straw as opposed to grain and relating this to crop processing stages (Harvey and Fuller 2005, 745).

Constraints on interpretation

While grasses, which include many staple crops (wheat, rice, millets) produce diagnostic phytoliths, not all plants produce silica bodies and fewer still create identifiable phytoliths. Furthermore, the same phytolith shape can be present in plants from different taxonomic groups, rendering identification problematic (Madella 1997, 294). In modern references it is possible to identify to genera and in some cases species but for archaeological material it is often possible to categorize only to sub family. For this study there is a potential methodological discrepancy between rice and millets. Rice produces distinctive morphologically-specific phytoliths in both leaves and husk;

less reference work has been done on millets and while they produce characteristic phytoliths in the husks, the leaves are difficult to identify. The majority of phytoliths in all samples are non-diagnostic, for example hairs. Taphonomy must also be considered, in particular differential preservation, the effects of dissolution by alkaline soils, destructive trampling and bioturbation. Finally there are issues of equifinality. There are many potential trajectories to arrive at an end state and consequently more than one possible interpretation of ratios produced by an assemblage.

Results

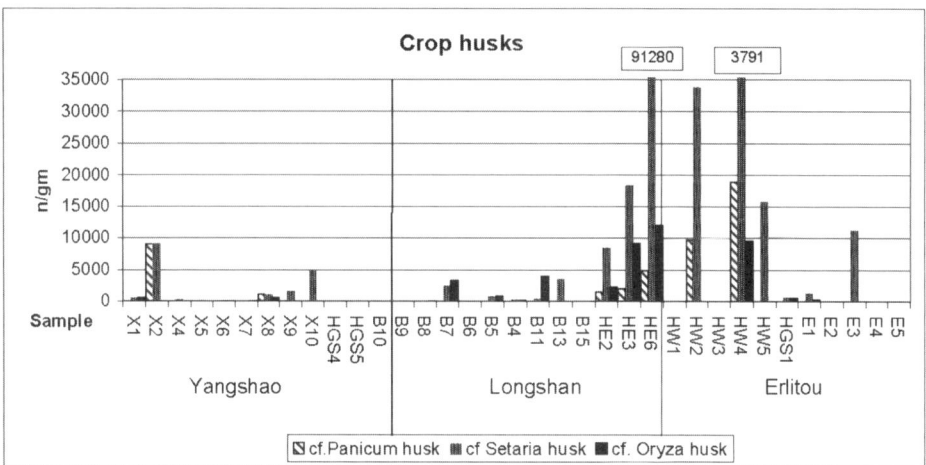

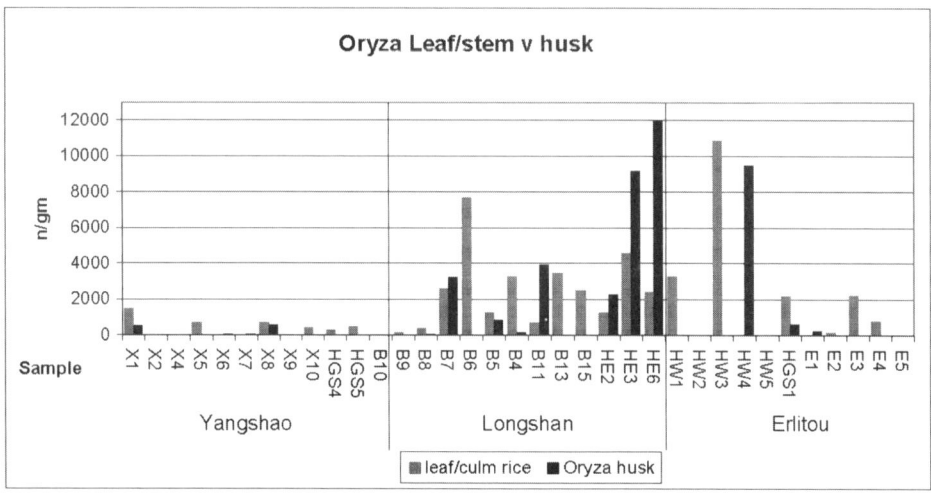

Figure 11.2. Charts of crop husk phytoliths and rice leaf/stem versus husk (sample key: X–Xipo, B–Baligang, H–Huizui, E– Erlitou).

Agricultural Crop Choices and Social Change

*Foxtail and Broomcorn (*Setaria italica and Panicum miliaceum*)*
The husk phytoliths follow the same broad pattern as the charred seeds in the macro remains from this region (Fuller and Zhang 2007; Lee and Bestel 2007; Lee *et al.* 2007). Foxtail seems predominant in the Yangshao at Xipo with broomcorn a secondary crop. No broomcorn was evident at Baligang during the Longshan. Both broomcorn and especially foxtail were abundant at Huizui in Longshan contexts. They have also been found in abundance at Huizui in Erlitou period contexts but no broomcorn and only one sample containing foxtail has been found in the Erlitou site samples.

*Rice (*Oryza sativa*)*
Rice is native to south China so was either grown as an introduced crop or traded in (Lee *et al.* 2007, 1088). Like foxtail, rice is more common towards the east and south. The densities of rice phytoliths over the Yangshao, Longshan and Erlitou periods show its presence in low concentrations throughout the Yangshao at Xipo and Huizui. There is a sharp increase at both Baligang and Huizui during the Longshan. However, of the Erlitou period samples, only one contains rice husks at Huizui West and one with low density at the Erlitou site. If the ratios of husk to leaf/stem are compared, higher proportions of straw are seen in many of the samples. This is not surprising as there are more leaves than husk on the plant. While they mostly correlate during the Yangshao, during the Longshan there are several samples that are either leaf/culm or husk. There is very poor correlation during the Erlitou Period at both Huizui and Erlitou with leaf/stems and husks present in different samples. This may suggest diversification in activities both within and between sites.

Discussion

Taking into consideration the limited data analysed so far, the results from these samples suggest changing agricultural cereal crop choices from the Yangshao to the Longshan and Erlitou Periods. How are they related to socio-economic development?

Economies are based on the procurement, processing, exchange and consumption of natural resources (Fuller and Stevens in press; Hastorf 1988; Simmons 1996). Vegetative material acquired by gathering and cultivation has long provided humans with food, fuel and technology. Plant remains are the direct results of these activities so can be linked to cultural and economic systems (Hastorf 1988, 119; Johannessen 1988, 145). Changes in social organization from egalitarian communal living to a more centralized hierarchy have been related to how labour was organized. As society became more integrated labour organization became more focused (Liu 2004; Liu and Chen 2003). One of the strengths of phytolith data is demonstrating broad patterning in plant remains. Comparing these patterns within samples from different time periods and sites should identify trends within the data that mirror changes in plant populations and human-plant interactions (Johannessen 1988, 149). Variables over time, such as crop choices, can indicate social change. Expansion or modification of cultivated land possibly showing specialization in the use of land resources and changes in technology, for example the development of rice paddies, might point to intensification and expansion (Netting 1974, 39). Storage is central to redistribution and trading. Large bell-shaped storage pits are ubiquitous in the region and the remains of their contents may provide insights to organization – for example how far along the processing path the crops are when stored – and from this it may be possible to infer information about relative quantities of labour needed to process and store the crop in that condition. In turn, this could inform on labour organization, whether it is small scale (e.g. a family unit), or indicative of large-scale mobilization. As harvest is a time of great labour demand, high densities of fully processed grain (phytoliths from husks) might suggest large groups mobilized to process the crop fully, whereas partially processed crops (phytoliths from leaves and stems) might point to smaller household use where processing is completed as the grain is needed (Harvey and Fuller 2005, 745)

During the Mid Neolithic, Yangshao early farming settlements were predominantly small, unstratified, often shifting villages (Chang 1986, 111). Charred seed evidence from Banpo suggests agriculture was practised alongside gathering (*ibid.*, 112). It is likely that labour was organized around kinship groups (*ibid.*, 119). The major crop in the Yellow River Valley seems to have been Foxtail; however, the uptake of rice can clearly be seen. The presence of rice leaf/stems at Xipo suggests it was being processed on-site, indicating paddies nearby. Environmental conditions had been stable and suitable for paddy farming for a long time before rice was adopted (Rosen 2007, 45) so the introduction of rice as a crop at this time could point to social motivation (possibly demographic pressure), developing social integration (Rosen 2007, 46), or the fact that rice was a only a relatively new domesticate (Fuller pers. comm.).

In the Longshan there was a distinctive change to permanent larger settlements with rammed earth defensive walls and two and three tiered hierarchies (Chang 1986, 248–9; Liu 2004, 115). Differentiation in settlement and household size and evidence of specialization in pottery, stone tools and textiles suggests more focussed labour organization (Liu 2004, 112). There are high densities of rice phytoliths in Longshan period contexts at Baligang, which is further south than the Yellow River Valley sites and increased levels at Huizui in the Yellow River Valley, although foxtail continues to be a significant crop here. This suggests a society capable of organized labour mobilization in order to build and maintain rice paddies. Rice leaf/stem phytoliths were present in all the Baligang samples suggesting crop-processing residues that include threshing and winnowing waste. This is mirrored at Huizui although here there are higher proportions of husk, which might point to storage of processed spikelets (hulled grains) (Figure 11.2 b). Foxtail husks dominate one sample from a large storage pit, suggesting foxtail was stored partially processed as whole grain and not dehusked until use. They are present alongside broomcorn in all the Longshan period samples from Huizui (Figure 11.2a), again indicating enough labour was mobilized at harvest time to process the crop to spikelets.

Broomcorn occurs in all cultural periods but in lower proportions than either foxtail or rice suggesting it was grown on a small scale possibly as a supplementary or buffer crop. Another possibility is that broomcorn is appearing as a foxtail crop weed but in the results so far there is a low correlation between broomcorn and foxtail husks (Figure 11.3a). The lack of evidence for broomcorn at Baligang during the Longshan may reflect the southern location in the Yangtze catchment, where conditions were possibly too warm and humid for broomcorn to thrive.

The Early Bronze Age Erlitou period witnessed the emergence of the first urban centre at Erlitou and distinct spatial differentiation within sites (Liu and Xu 2007, 886). The cooler, arid climatic conditions meant the environment had become more suitable for dry land crops such as millets. This is borne out by the predominance of foxtail and, to a lesser extent, broomcorn in the Huizui samples. The Erlitou period samples from Huizui demonstrate a general increase in millet densities and fall in rice. At Erlitou the samples contain few husk phytoliths, possibly suggesting grain was being traded in from outside, a potential response to decreasing available agricultural land and the development of specialized craft industries and trade at Huizui (stone tools) and Erlitou (bronze and ceramics), or else being processed fully to cleaned grain. However, as the Erlitou samples are from a palace area, the phytoliths are not representative of the city as a whole. Rice appears in very low densities. At Huizui the densities are higher with a distinct contrast between husk and leaf/stem samples. The comparatively high densities of leaf/stem at Huizui West point to early processing taking place on site (Harvey and Fuller 2005, 745). This does not correspond with the very low ratios for husks supporting the possibility that rice was being traded out.

Conclusion

While the relationship between social development and crop choices is complex, the data from the plant remains from these four sites show some interesting patterns. The evidence from these phytolith assemblages suggests that cereal crop choices changed over the three cultural periods. The most significant factor seems to have been the uptake and expansion of rice agriculture. The organization and mobilization of labour needed to farm rice corresponds with the social development seen in the construction of large rammed-earth walls, craft specialization and the emergence of tiered hierarchies. Despite environmental changes from warm, wet and marshy to cool and arid with less land available, rice seems to have maintained its importance at least as a secondary crop suggesting its possible role as an elite product.

Acknowledgements

This project was funded by the AHRC and fieldwork was made possible by Li Liu and Xingcan Chen.

References

An, C., Feng, Z. and Barton, L. 2006. 'Dry or humid? Mid Holocene humidity changes in arid and semi-arid China', *Quaternary Science Reviews* **25**, 351–61.

An, C., Feng, Z. and Tang, L. 2004. 'Environmental change and cultural response between 8000 and 4000 cal. yr BP in the western Loess Plateau, northwest China', *Journal of Quaternary Science* **19**, 529–35.

An, Z., Porter, S.C., Kutzbach, J.E., Wu, X., Wang, S., Liu, X., Li, X. and Zhou, W. 2000. 'Asynchronous Holocene optimum of the East Asian monsoon', *Quaternary Science Reviews* **19**, 743–62.

Chang, K.C. 1986. *The Archaeology of Ancient China* (New Haven and London).

Chi, Y., Kong, Z., Wang, S., Tang, L., Yao, T., Zhao, X., Zhang, P. and Shi, S.1993. 'Mid Holocene climates and environments in China', *Global and Planetary Change* **7**, 219–33.

Dykoski, C.A., Lawrence Edwards, R., Cheng, H., Yuan, D., Cai, Y., Zhang, M., Lin, Y., Qing, J., An, Z. and Revenaugh, J. 2005. 'A high-resolution, absolute-dated Holocene and deglacial Asian monsoon record from Dongge Cave, China', *Earth and Planetary Science Letters* **233**, 71–86.

Feng, Z.D., An, C., Tang, L.Y. and Jull, A.J.T. 2004. 'Stratigraphic evidence of a Megahumid climate between 10,000 and 4000 years B.P. in the western part of the Chinese Loess Plateau', *Global and Planetary Change* **43**, 145–55

Feng, Z.D., An, C. and Wang, H.B. 2006. 'Holocene climatic and environmental changes in the arid and semi-arid areas of China: a review', *The Holocene* **16**, 119–30.

Ford, A. 2004. 'Ground stone tool production at Huizui, China: an analysis of a manufacturing site in the Yilou River Basin', *Bulletin of Indo-Pacific Prehistory Association* **24**, 71–7.

Fuller, D.Q., Ling, Q. and Harvey, E. 2007. 'A critical assessment of early agriculture in East Asia, with the emphasis in Lower Yangtze rice domestication', *Pradghara Journal of the Uttar Pradesh State Archaeology Department* (special issue), 1–26.

Fuller, D.Q. and Stevens, C. in press. 'Agriculture and the development of complex societies: an archaeobotanical agenda', in Fairbairn, A. and Weiss, E. (eds) *Ethnobotanist of Distant Pasts: Papers in Honour of Gordon Hillman* (Oxford).

Fuller, D.Q. and Zhang, H. 2007. 'A preliminary report of the survey of archaeobotany of the upper Ying Valley (Henan Province)' in School of Archaeology and Museology, Peking University and Henan Provincial Institute of Cultural Relics and Archaeology (ed.) *Dengfeng wangchenggang yizhi de faxian yu yanjiu (2002–2005) [Archaeological Discovery and Research at the Wangchenggang Site in Dengfeng (2002–2005)]* [in English & Chinese] (Zhengzhou), 916–58.

Harvey, E. and Fuller, D.Q. 2005. 'Investigating crop processing using phytolith analysis', *Journal of Archaeological Science* **32**, 739–52.

Hastorf, C.A. 1988. 'The use of palaeoethnobotanic data in studies of crop production, processing and consumption', in Hastorf, C.A. and Popper, V.S. (eds) *Current Palaeoethnobotany: Analytical Methods and Cultural Interpretations of Archaeological Plant Remains* (Chicago), 119–44.

Herzschuh, U., Tarasov, P., Wunnemann, B. and Hartmann, K. 2004. 'Holocene vegetation and climate of the Alashan Plateau, NW China, reconstructed from pollen data', *Palaeogeography, Palaeoclimatology, Palaeoecology* **211**, 1–7.

Jiang, Q. and Zhang, J. 1998. 'Phytolith evidence for rice cultivation during prehistoric periods at Baligang site of Baizhuang, Dengzhou City, Henan Province', *Acta Scientarium Naturalium Universitatis Pekinensis* **34**, 66–71.

Johannessen, S. 1988. 'Plant remains and culture change: are palaeoethnobotanical data better than we think?', in Hastorf, C.A. and Popper, V.S. (eds) *Current Palaeoethnobotany: Analytical Methods and Cultural Interpretations of Archaeological Plant Remains* (Chicago), 145–66.

Lee, G.-A. and Bestel, S. 2007. 'Contextual analysis of plant remains at the Erlitou-period Huizui site, Henan, China', *Indo-Pacific Prehistory Association Bulletin* 27, 49–60.

Lee, G.-A., Crawford, G., Liu, L. and Chen, X. 2007. 'Plants and people from the early Neolithic to the Shang periods in North China', *Proceedings of the National Academy of Sciences* 104, 1087–92.

Lee, Y.K. 2004. 'Control strategies and polity competition in the lower Yi-Luo Valley, North China', *Journal of Anthropological Archaeology* 23, 172–95.

Liu, L. 1996. 'Settlement patterns, chiefdom, variability and the development of early states in north China', *Journal of Anthropological Archaeology* 15, 237–88.

Liu, L. 2004. *The Chinese Neolithic: Trajectories to Early States* (Cambridge).

Liu, L. and Chen, X. 2003. *State Formation in Early China* (London).

Liu, L., Chen, X., Lee, Y.K., Wright, H. and Rosen, A. 2004. 'Settlement patterns and development of social complexity in the Yilou region, North China', *Journal of Field Archaeology* 29, 75–100.

Liu, L. and Xu, H. 2007. 'Rethinking Erlitou: legend, history and Chinese archaeology', *Antiquity* 81, 886–901.

Lu, T. 2002. 'A green foxtail millet (Foxtail *viridis*) cultivation experiment in the middle Yellow River Valley', *Asian perspectives* 41, 1–14.

Ma, X. 2005. *Emergent Social complexity in the Yangshao Culture: Analyses of Settlement Patterns and Faunal Remains from Lingbao, Western Henan, China* (Oxford).

Madella, M. 1997. 'Phytolith analysis from the Indus Valley site of Kot Diji Sind, Pakistan', in Sinclair, A., Slater, E. and Gowlet, J. (eds) *Archaeological Sciences 1995: Proceedings of a conference on the application of scientific techniques to the study of archaeology* (Oxford), 294–302.

Maher, B.A. and Hu, M. 2006. 'A high resolution record of Holocene rainfall variations from the western Chinese Loess Plateau: antiphase behaviour of the African/ Indian and East Asian summer monsoons', *The Holocene* 16, 309–19.

Netting, R.M. 1974. 'Agrarian Ecology', *Annual Review of Anthropology* 3, 21–56.

Netting, R.M. 1993. *Smallholders, Householders: Farm Families and the Ecology of Intensive Sustainable Agriculture* (Stanford).

Rosen, A.M. 2007. 'The role of environmental change in the development of complex societies in China: a study from the Huizui site', *Indo-Pacific Prehistory Association Bulletin* 27, 39–48.

Simmons, I.G. 1996. *Changing the Face of the Earth* (Oxford).

Underhill, A.P. 1997. 'Current issues in Chinese Neolithic archaeology', *Journal of World Prehistory* 11, 103–60.

Wu, W. and Liu, T. 2004. 'Possible role of the "Holocene Event 3" on the collapse of Neolithic cultures around the Central Plain of China', *Quaternary International* 117, 153–66.

Xiao, J., Xu, Q., Nakamura, T., Yang, X., Liang, W. and Inouchi, Y. 2004. 'Holocene vegetation variation in the Daihai Lake region of north-central China: a direct indication of the Asian monsoon climatic history', *Quaternary Science Reviews* 23, 1669–79.

Shorter Contributions

The Dynamics of Anglo-Saxon Fish Consumption

Rebecca Reynolds,
University of Nottingham

Industrial marine fishing and widespread fish consumption appear to have begun around 1000 AD; prior to this there is little evidence that marine fish were eaten regularly, especially outside urban contexts (Barrett *et al.* 2004). However, recent excavations of the rural, possibly thegnly (aristocratic), settlement at Bishopstone in East Sussex have yielded substantial quantities of marine fish remains in deposits dating between the eighth and tenth centuries. This assemblage is highly interesting given the relative dearth of fish consumption in the period, raising the possibility that marine fishing may have been instigated by rural elites rather than being the result of wider economic developments associated with urban growth, as has been suggested by Barrett *et al.* (2004).

The Assemblage

Using a rapid recording strategy, based on a small suite of fish elements, 2448 specimens were identified, with 17 different taxa represented. Surprisingly, very few freshwater species were identified (only 15 cyprinid vertebrae and a few bones of perch, *Perca fluviatilis*), the assemblage being dominated by migratory and marine species. With

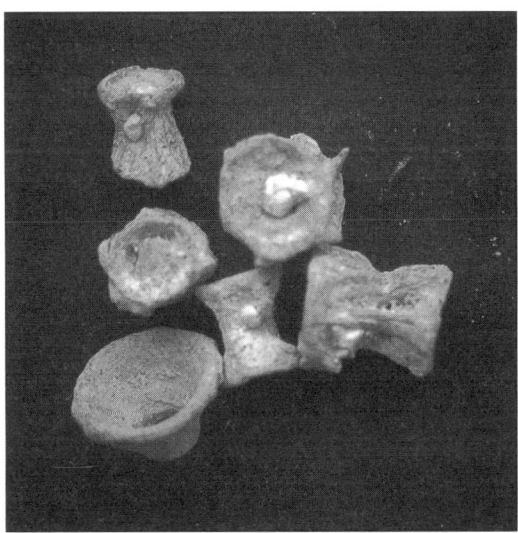

Figure 12.1. Digested unidentifiable fish vertebrae.

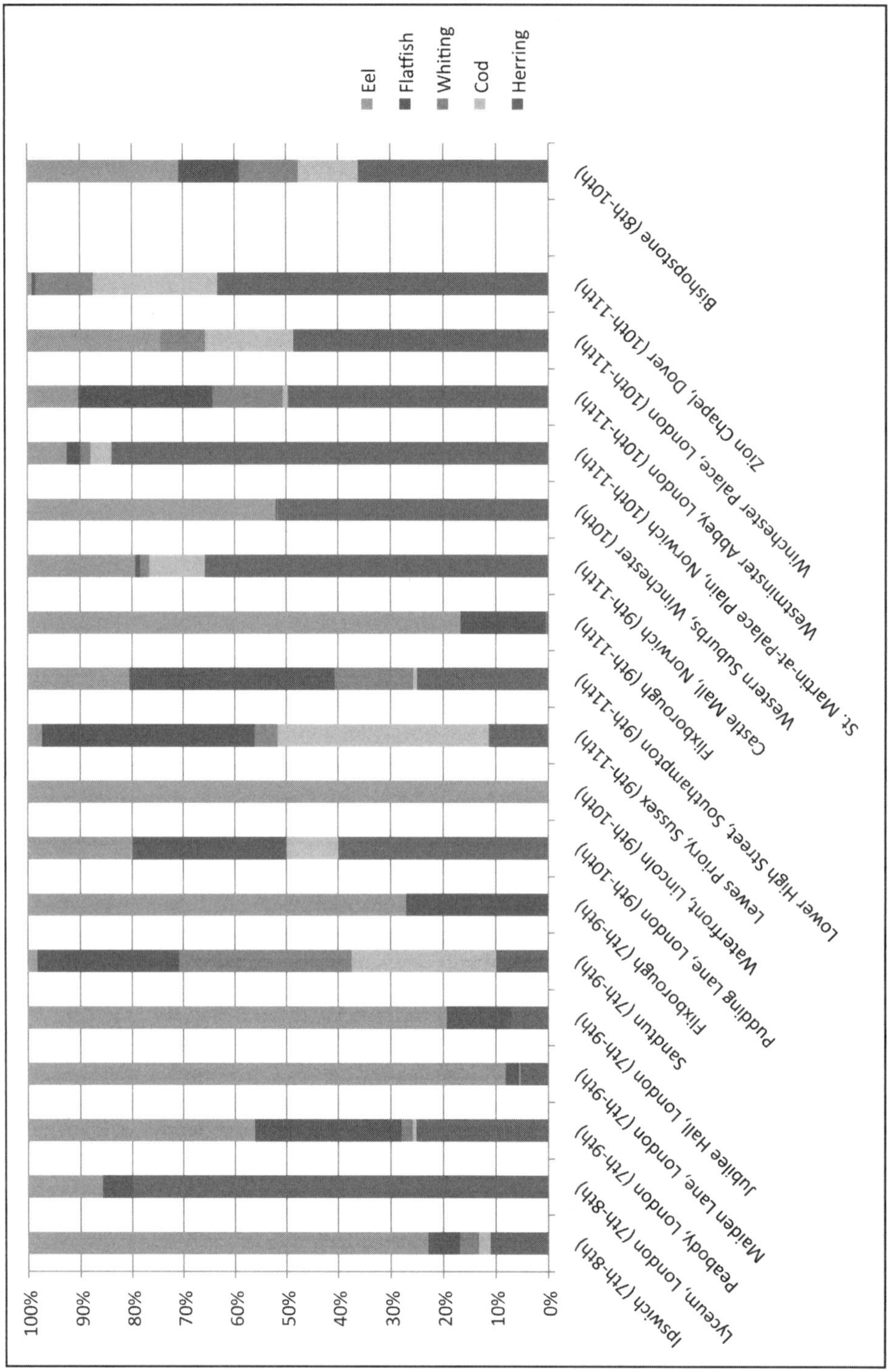

The Dynamics of Anglo-Saxon Fish Consumption

Figure 12.2. Relative frequencies of herring, cod, whiting, flatfish and eel from different sites. For references see Reynolds (in prep.).

the exception of one tentatively-identified salmonid bone, eel (*Anguilla anguilla*) were the only migratory taxon. Of the marine species, herring (*Clupea harrengus*) was most abundant, followed by cod (*Gadus morhua*), whiting (*Merlangius merlangus*), Atlantic mackerel *(Scombrus scombrus)* and scad *(Trachurus trachurus)*. The presence of rays (Rajidae) was noted from the high numbers of dermal denticles and ossified vertebrae.

Vertebrae account for most of the fish remains; however cranial elements, such as maxilla and pre-maxilla, were present in sufficient quantities to conclude that fish were brought to the site complete. The only possible exception is herring, for which only vertebrae were found, perhaps suggesting that the heads were removed elsewhere. Many of the eel and herring vertebrae, especially those from the cess pit deposits, were crushed and digested, presumably having been eaten and excreted by people (Figure 12.1). There seems to be a division in the composition of deposits, some being dominated by eel, herring and small whiting vertebrae whilst others contained the remains of bigger fish such as cod, flatfish, rays and scad. Those dominated by the bigger fish also contained higher quantities of large mammals and it seems possible that these variations reflect differences in the deposits' formation: latrine versus kitchen and table waste.

All the fish present could have been locally caught, either in the estuary or along the coast using a variety of weirs, lines and nets. Though no traps have been found or are mentioned in the Domesday Book, this does not exclude their existence. Eels could easily have been caught in wicker baskets or traps stretched across the river to catch them when they swim upstream as elvers or downstream as adults (Locker n.d.). Flounder (*Platichthys flessus*) will often come up estuaries where they can be caught using 'kiddles' or 'sea hedges' which trap the fish as it comes inshore with the tide (Locker n.d.). Cod and whiting could have been caught inshore, where they often venture, using a line, while herring and mackerel would have required the use of a floating net (Locker 1987).

Bishopstone in its wider context
Barrett *et al.* (2004, 627) suggested that, prior to the eleventh century, marine fishing may have been a preserve of the elite but, up to now, there has been little evidence to explore the possibility more fully. Bishopstone is clearly a high-status rural site and so has the potential to address this knowledge gap. While there is no definite phasing for Bishopstone, AMS dating suggests that it was occupied between the eighth and tenth centuries, prior to the so-called 'Fish Event Horizon' (Barrett *et al.* 2004).

The significance of the Bishopstone assemblage is highlighted when it is compared with data from other contemporary sites. For instance, marine fish remains are rare from Middle Saxon (seventh to mid-ninth-century) sites, and where they have been recovered in quantity – e.g. from coastal and 'urban' sites such as *Sandtun* in Kent (Hamilton-Dyer 2002) and Ipswich in Suffolk (Locker and Jones 1985) – the species diversity is small. Large deposits of fish remains were also found at Flixborough (Lincolnshire), though here only a small number of marine species were represented (Dobney *et al.* 2007). Fish remains are more common at Late Anglo-Saxon (mid-ninth to mid-eleventh-century) urban sites such as Westminster Abbey (Locker 1997), Southampton (Hamilton-Dyer 1997), Winchester (Coy in press) and several sites from Norwich (Locker 1987; 1994; Locker forthcoming).

The Bishopstone assemblage has characteristics (e.g. large quantities of eel bones) typical of Middle Saxon assemblages, along with traits (large quantities of marine fish) common to assemblages from Late Anglo-Saxon urban sites. It stands apart from other assemblages by the diversity and quantity of marine species it contains, demonstrating that, on this site at least, consumption of marine fish was being practised well before the 'Fish Event Horizon'. Further research will help to ascertain whether other elite sites demonstrate similar evidence for an early uptake of fish-eating. If this is the case it may suggest that elite dietary practices were responsible for driving the 'Fish Event Horizon'.

Acknowledgements

I am extremely grateful to Dr James Barrett and Dr Heide Hüster-Plogmann for teaching me my first fish identifying skills. Many thanks are due to Alison Locker and Sheila Hamilton-Dyer for supplying many of their unpublished reports. I am also very grateful to Dr Naomi Sykes and Dr Claire Newton for their comments.

References

Barrett, J.H., Locker, A.M. and Roberts, C.M. 2004. "Dark Age Economics' revisited: the English fish bone evidence AD 600–1600', *Antiquity* 78, 618–36.

Coy, J. in press. 'Late Saxon and medieval animal bone from the Western Suburbs', in Serjeanston, D. and Reehs, H. (eds) *Food, Craft and Status in Medieval Winchester: The Evidence from the Suburbs and City Defences* (Winchester).

Dobney, K., Jaques, D., Barrett, J. and Johnstone, C. 2007. *Farmers, Monks and Aristocrats: the Environmental Archaeology of Anglo-Saxon Flixborough. Excavations at Flixborough Volume 3,* (Oxford).

Hamlton-Dyer, S. 1997. *The Lower High Street Project, Southampton: The Faunal Remains.* Unpublished report.

Hamilton-Dyer, S. 2002. 'Bird and fish remains' in Gardiner M., Cross R., Macpherson-Grant N. and Riddler I. (eds) 'Continental trade and non-urban ports in Middle Anglo-Saxon England: excavations at Sandtun, West Hythe, Kent', *Archaeological Journal* 158, 255–61.

Locker, A. 1987. 'The fish remains', in Ayers, B. (ed.) *Excavations at St. Martin-at-Palace Plain, Norwich, 1981* (Norwich).

Locker, A. 1994. 'Fish bones', in Ayers, B.S. (ed.) *Excavations at Fishergate, Norwich, 1985,* (Norwich).

Locker, A. 1997. 'The fish bones', in Mills, P. (ed.) 'Excavations at the dorter undercroft, Westminster Abbey', *Transactions of the London and Middlesex Archaeological Society* 46, 111–13.

Locker, A. Forthcoming. 'The Anglo-Saxon period IV zoological and botanical evidence', in Albarella, U., Beech, M., Locker, A., Moreno-Garcia, M., Mulville, J., Curl, J. and Shepherd-Pescu, E. (eds) *Norwich Castle: Excavations and Historical Survey 1987–98. Part III: A Zooarchaeological Study,* (Norwich).

Locker, A. n.d. *Milk Street, London: The Fish Bones.* Unpublished report.

Locker, A. and Jones, A. 1985. *Ipswich: the fish remains. AML Report 4578,* (London).

Reynolds, R. In preparation. *The Fish Remains from Bishopstone.*

Poor Man's Silver? The Role of Pewter in Roman Britain: A Collection in The British Museum

Lindsey Smith,
University of Reading and the British Museum

This brief paper will introduce on-going research into a small collection of Romano-British pewter vessels, currently housed in The British Museum (see Website 1), that offers the opportunity to understand the relationships people had with pewter. The Museum's collection, which has been growing since 1844, contains just over one hundred Romano-British pewter vessels and this is the first time it has been fully researched or published. The majority of items are bowls, platters, plates, cups, jugs and ingots but little is known about their use and function in the Roman period.

Pewter vessels were apparently particularly favoured in Roman Britain, with just a small number being known from the continent, mostly from burials in Holland, Belgium and France (Beagrie 1989). The majority of British finds come from south of the Fosse Way (see Figure 13.1) with concentrations around the Fens and the Mendips, areas thought to be the main production centres (Beagrie 1989; Wedlake 1958). This distribution suggests that pewter was a material solely manufactured in Britain for a British market. Emergence of the pewter industry is difficult to date due to the durable nature of pewter vessels, i.e. they do not break easily, can be repaired and so have a long lifespan. It is conceivable that pewter was being manufactured throughout the Roman period; however, a peak in deposition, and probably production, certainly occurred in the later Roman period: most pewter vessels have been recovered from late Roman hoards dating to the later third and fourth centuries, the earliest examples dating to about AD 250 (Wedlake 1958). The shape and forms of the bowl, plates, spoons and cup purported from the stream bed of the Walbrook, London suggested a mid first century date for manufacture (Merrifield 1969, 162–3); however, X-ray fluorescence analysis demonstrated that these vessels were actually either tin or lead (Jones 1983, 52–4). Whilst this challenges the theory that pewterware was manufactured in *Londinium* before the mid-third century, it does suggest that a tin industry existed in the Walbrook area around AD 155, producing tableware items that were later copied into pewter (Jones 1983, 52).

Pewter use
A common interpretation is that Roman pewter vessels were functional, utilitarian pieces which served as the typical 'dining accoutrement' of wealthy villa owners of the third and fourth centuries (Brown 1973, 201–4), being a 'cheap substitute for costly silver' (Wedlake 1958, 85). Certainly the shapes and detailing of some vessels in the

collection match shapes contemporary in silver and bronze from the first, second and third centuries; for example a pewter platter from Coldham Common resembles the silver dish from Mildenhall (Henig 1995, 132) and the square dish from Icklingham is a form similar to the silver Mileham Dish (both in the British Museum). Interlocking triangles appear on the underside of a flanged bowl from Lakenheath and the same motif decorates the central roundel of the fluted silver bowl from Mildenhall (Painter 1977, fig 31). Similarly, there are vessels within the British Museum's collection that fit the tableware assumptions with graffiti referring to what may be personal ownership: these also provide the opportunity to discuss issues of literacy, early iconography and epigraphy. Distribution of pewter vessels also tends to support this idea, with the majority of finds appearing in what is believed to be the 'civil' zone of Roman Britain south of the Fosse Way (Peal 1967, 22; see Figure 13.1).

However, some finds have been recovered from areas not typically associated with high Roman villa density, such as Suffolk, Norfolk and the Fens in East Anglia. Indeed pewter vessels are often found in association with wet or watery places, for instance wells (such as those from Silchester and Brislington) and in old river beds: the alluvium deposit of the Thames at Shepperton and Welney (Cambs). We have, therefore, to

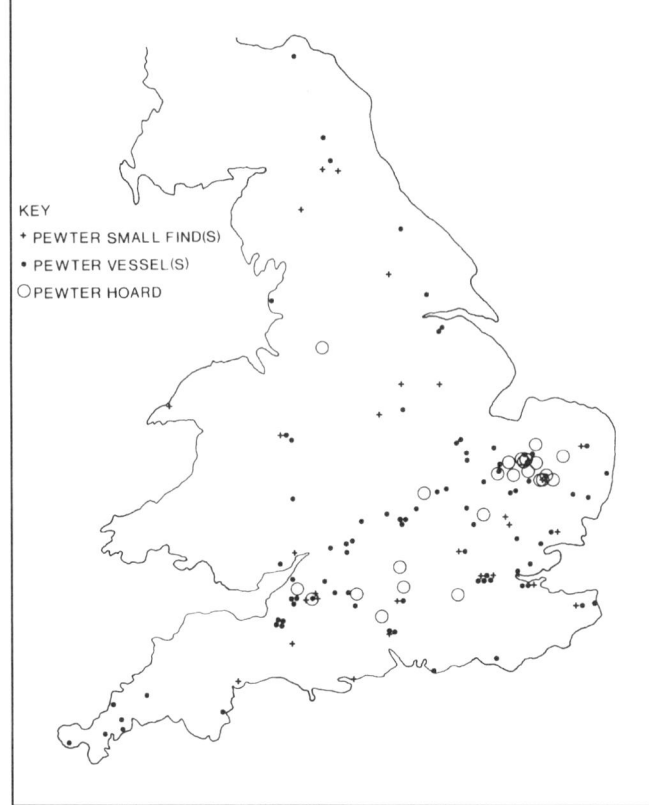

Figure 13.1. Distribution map of pewter small finds, vessels and hoards (reproduced from Beagrie 1989, 177).

consider the possibility that pewter vessels were deliberately buried as ritual or votive dedications (Beagrie 1989, 178–9; Poulton and Scott 1993). As with lead, perhaps pewter was specifically chosen for ritualistic items due to the chthonic nature of the material (Tomlin 1988, 81).

Another interesting trait of Romano-British pewterware is that some specimens appear to have been 'ritually pierced' or 'deliberately holed'. A number of pewter vessels in the collection bear 'stab' or 'puncture' wounds that would render them useless as 'plates', 'bowls' and 'jugs'. The 'ritual killing' of objects as sacrifice or as votives is well attested in Roman Britain. For example, smashed pots and miniature implements, tools and 'bent' weapons have been recovered from the Roman Temple sites of Uley, Verulamium and Woodeaton (Henig 1984, 148–152). At Silchester, a pewter flagon demonstrating a circular hole just above the base was recovered from a well shaft that had been sealed by an ogham-inscribed baluster stone column. The hole is interpreted as deliberate, rendering the vessel useless in terms of its perceived primary function; to hold liquids (Fulford and Timby 2001, 295). It is possible that, as with Iron Age and Romano-British pottery, the British Museum pewter vessels were 'ritual killed' as part of a ritual of deposition (Fulford *et al.* 2000; Hill 1995) and the motivation for the creation and subsequent damage of the pewter plates is certainly worthy of further investigation.

Religious association?

A number of vessels in the collection bear the 'Chi-Rho' (a symbol used by Christians – formed by the first two letters of the Greek word for 'Christ') that is known from silver plate hoards such as Mildenhall and Water Newton (see Figure 13.2). It is not inconceivable that the large pewter platters may have been used in ceremonial feasting (Heing 1995, 133). The vessels may also represent a donation to the church as liturgical plate suggestive of pewter being substituted for silver by the less prosperous Romano-British congregation and thus allowing those less wealthy or powerful to participate

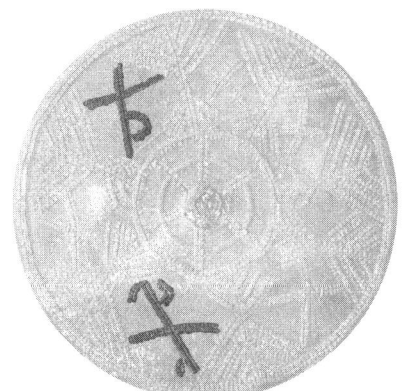

Figure 13.2. Pewter Plate from the collection bearing the (hidden) Chi-Rho (drawn by Stephen Crummy, © Trustees of The British Museum).

in religious activities. The location of the graffiti or decoration on the vessels may be significant, for example whether the inscription could be seen or hidden from sight under the rim, or were images hidden if food or offerings were placed within the vessel.

Comparisons with other materials

It is already clear that the British Museum pewter vessels exhibit forms comparable with vessels in ceramics, glass or silver from Britain and on the Continent. For instance, small hemispherical bowls with broad rims and low pedestal foots are analogous to the small samian cup 'Form 35'. A number of pewter plates bear low relief decoration, often a rosette in the centre and bead-and-reel around a flat rim that is reminiscent of the detailing on bronze and silver vessels. Advances in this area of research will have the potential to address wider social, economic and art-historical influences; for example the relationship of vessel form to contemporary ceramics and silver vessels.

Conclusion

This brief review of Romano-British pewter vessels has shown that their traditional interpretation, as a tableware, is perhaps too simplistic, especially given that pewter is a soft material (with a high lead content) that does not lend itself for use at the table. Instead, pewter vessels appear to have carried far greater social and religious significance. Comprehension of this significance may be achieved only through detailed study of the objects and the contexts in which they were found. By cataloguing vessel shape and form, wear marks and inscriptions it will be possible to compare pewter data with those for other ranges of artefacts (ceramics, glass and metals) across regions and continents. Ultimately it is hoped that studies of the kind I am currently undertaking on the British Museum's collection will provide a stimulus for wider debates concerning how we can study value-laden artefacts.

Acknowledgements

I wish to thank Professor Mike Fulford and Dr Hella Eckardt from Reading University and Dr Richard Hobbs from The British Museum for their encouragement and help during this ongoing research. Dr Martin Henig and Craig Gibbin for their enthusiasm and support and The British Museum and the Arts and Humanities Research Council who are funding the project. I am also very grateful to Dr Neil Beagrie and the Trustees of the British Museum for allowing me to reproduce their images.

References

Beagrie, N. 1989. 'The Romano-British pewter industry', *Britannia* 10, 169–191.
Brown, D. 1973. 'A Roman pewter hoard from Appleford, Berks', *Oxoniensia* 38, 184–206.
Fulford, M. and Timby, J. 2001. 'Timing devices, fermentation vessels, 'ritual piercings? A consideration of deliberately 'holed' pots from Silchester and elsewhere', *Britannia* 32, 293–7.
Fulford, M., Handley, M., and Clarke, A. 2000. 'An early date for Ogham: the Silchester Ogham stone rehabilitated', *Medieval Archaeology* 44, 1–23.
Henig, M. 1984. *Religion in Roman Britain* (London).
Henig, M. 1995. *The Art of Roman Britain* (London).
Hill, J.D. 1995. *Ritual and Rubbish in the Iron Age of Wessex: a study on the formation of a specific archaeological record.* BAR 242 (Oxford).
Jones, C.E.E. 1983. 'A review of Roman lead-alloy material recovered from the Walbrook Valley in the City of London', *Transactions of the London and Middlesex Archaeological Society* 34, 49–59.
Merrifield, R. 1969. *Roman London* (London).
Painter, K.S. 1977. *The Mildenhall Treasure: Roman Silver from East Anglia* (London).
Peal, C.A. 1967. 'Romano-British pewter plates and dishes', *Proceedings of the Cambridge Antiquarian Society* 60, 19–37.
Poulton, R. and Scott, E. 1993. 'The hoarding, deposition and use of pewter in Roman Britain', *Theoretical Roman Archaeology: first conference proceedings* (Aldershot) 115–32.
Tomlin, R.S.O. 1988. 'The curse tablets', in B. Cunliffe (ed) *The Temple of Sulis Minerva at Bath. Vol 2. The Finds from the Sacred Spring* (Oxford), 9–21.
Wedlake, W.J. 1958. *Excavations at Camerton, Somerset* (Camerton).

Website 1. http://www.britishmuseum.org/research/research_projects/pewter_hoards.aspx

Eat Drink and Influence People:
The Cutlers' Company Annual Feast

Joan Unwin,
University of Sheffield

In 1624, the cutlers of Sheffield applied to Parliament for an Act of Incorporation to regulate their trade. Since at least the end of the thirteenth century, knives had been made in and around Sheffield, eventually coming under the control of the manorial courts of the Lords of Hallamshire, the powerful Earls of Shrewsbury. With the death of last resident lord in 1619, it was necessary to continue control over the numbers of apprentices and times of work, which had been administered by the local court. The Act of Incorporation established the Company of Cutlers in Hallamshire, with an annually elected Company of thirty-three members led by the Master Cutler. Every year, on or around the feast of St Bartholomew in August, a new Company was elected; the year's accounts checked; the Master installed; a church service was held and finally, the new Company had a dinner.

For almost every year since 1625, the Company has held a dinner (later to be called The Feast). Beginning as a private dinner in a local inn, the occasion increased in importance as the seventeenth century wore on, when leading townspeople and the local gentry were invited. The Company had its own hall from 1638, on a site opposite the parish church (now the cathedral) and had room to accommodate its guests to dinner. Without Parliamentary representation, the Sheffield cutlers had to rely on the influence of local JPs and landowners to make their voice heard in London and inviting them to its feast became an accepted policy. The Company successfully lobbied against the local enforcement of the Hearth Tax on cutlers in the 1670s and 1680s and, in the mid-eighteenth century, canvassed support for a Bill to improve the River Don for transporting goods into and out of Sheffield.

In his memoirs, Sir John Reresby, a local JP, recorded for 28 August, 1680:

> I went with my wife and family to the Cutlers' Feast at Sheffield, with some neighbours. I took with me the number of nearly thirty horse. The Master and Wardens, attended by an infinite crowd, met me at the entrance into the town with music and hautboys. I alighted from my coach, and went afoot with the Master to the Hall, where we had an extraordinary dinner; but it was at the charge of the Corporation of Cutlers. (MacDonald 1997, 227)

The Cutlers' Company Annual Feast

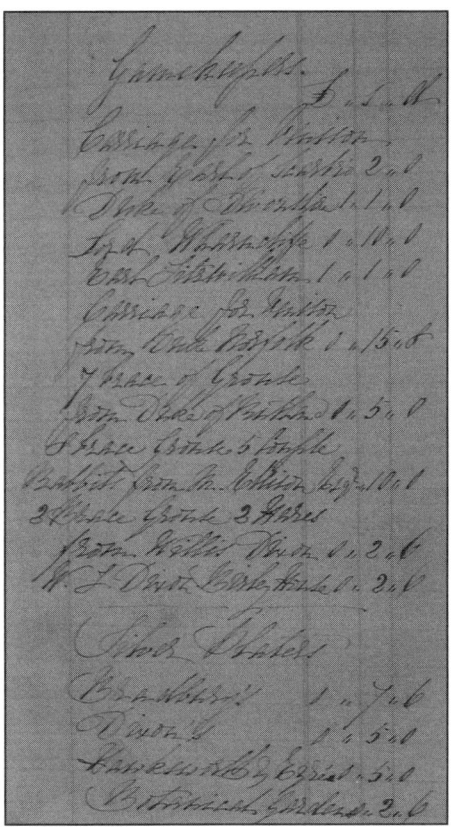

Figure 14.1. Page from the accounts of Thomas Moulson, Master Cutler, 1854.

Apart from a few comments on early feasts, the only other source of information about them, until the nineteenth century, is the Masters' accounts. The first hall was demolished and a second hall was built on the same site in 1723 and the account books record its fitting out and furnishing. For instance, chairs, tables, dozens of knives, cooking equipment and jelly glasses were purchased. Every year, the feast preparations included refurbishing the hall, cleaning the linen, knives and pewter, and repairing tables, chairs and cooking pans. Although additional purchases were made, such as more tablecloths, mugs, pitchers and plates, the accounts show the Company also had to hire trestle tables, glasses and spoons from local inns for the feast, a necessity which continued into the twentieth century, when items were hired from department stores and silver manufacturers.

There are only a few hints about what food was on the menu at the early feasts. As well as being invited to the feast, many local landowners sent their gamekeepers to the hall with gifts of venison, grouse, hares, etc. The gamekeepers were often 'treated' at alehouses or given a hunting knife for their efforts. In 1854, Thomas Moulson, the Master Cutler kept details of his feast and under the heading 'Gamekeepers', a total of £4.9s.8d. (£4.48p) was paid for the carriage of game.

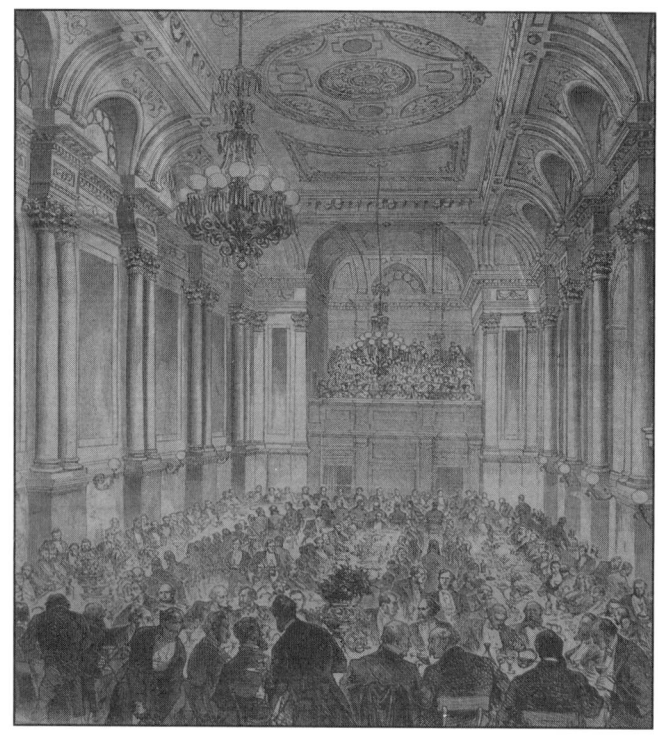

*Figure 14.2. The Cutlers' Feast of Mark Firth, Master Cutler in 1867, in the new Great Banqueting Hall (*London Illustrated News, *November, 1867).*

Venison was sent by the Earl of Scarbrough, the Dukes of Devonshire and Norfolk, Lord Wharncliffe and Earl Fitzwilliam and other guests sent eight brace of grouse, five couple of rabbits, two brace of grouse and two hares. Silver manufacturers, Bradbury's and James Dixon's, loaned table silver and 2s. 6d. (12p) was paid to Sheffield's Botanical Gardens for flowers.

From the mid-nineteenth century, with the expansion of steel manufacture in Sheffield, the Cutlers' Company amended the qualifications for membership in 1860 to include the steel and edge tool manufacturers. The Company had rebuilt its hall in 1832 and when the steel manufacturers became members and Masters, the hall was extended in 1866 to include an impressive new banqueting hall. From then on, the Company used the feast to reach the ears of people in the Armed Forces, the War Department and other government officials in order to promote the local firms manufacturing steel, armament and tools.

The archive of the Master Cutler, Charles Belk, contains the invitations, letters, programme and notes for his feast in September, 1885 and show his efforts to secure his principal guests and organise the seating plan for 410 guests, some of whom did not reply until the day before. Belk's feast menu is typical of period, with large number of courses and wines being served. His guest list included Lord Randolph Churchill, Secretary of State for India as his principal speaker plus Mr. C. B. Stuart-Wortley, M.P. for Sheffield Hallam, who was Under Secretary for the Home Department and Mr. B.

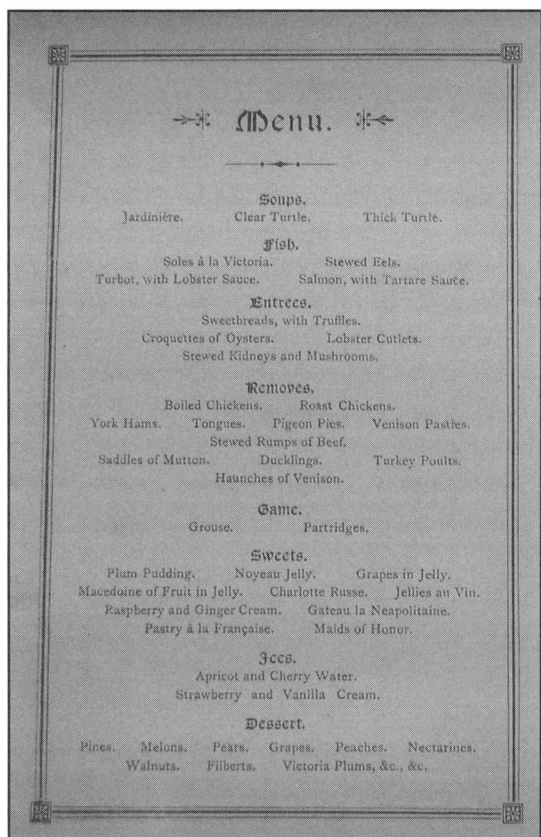

Figure 14.3. Menu for the Feast of Charles Belk, Master Cutler, 1885.

Ashmead-Bartlett, Civil Lord of the Admiralty. Continuing the tradition of inviting the local nobility and landowners the Dukes of Norfolk and of Rutland and the Earls of Scarbrough and of Wharncliffe were also invited. Also on the guest list was the United States Ambassador, Mr E.J. Phelps.

Until the middle of the twentieth century, the members of the Cutlers' Company were the major employers in Sheffield and what they said and did impinged on the lives of the local community. From the middle of the nineteenth century, the feast was covered by the press, both local and national, and the speeches were reported in detail. These reports of the speeches by the principal guests and the Masters' responses ensured that the concerns of the Sheffield manufacturers reached a wide audience, so it was vital that the feast could successfully highlight the steel and cutlery industry. As well as talking to their guests, the Masters arranged visits to factories for the following day. It is not known when this tradition began, but in Charles Belk's archive there is a note from Stephen Buridge of John Brown's Atlas Steel and Iron Works offering the factory for a visit, including a chance to see armour plate being cast. These works visits were intended to impress visitors who had the power to order steel and armaments from

Sheffield firms. In 1904, Master Cutler George Hall took his guests on a comprehensive tour of Hadfield's Hecla Works. His principal guest was Major General Sir Leslie Rundle. In 1906, William Fawcett Osborn invited Lord Tweedmouth, First Lord of the Admiralty and Baron Komura, the Japanese Ambassador. The guest lists continued to include high-ranking military men and members of the government with interests in the armed forces, trade and foreign affairs. For instance, in 1913, Thomas Ward invited Sir John Simon MP, the Attorney General; Admiral Sir Wilmot Fawkes; Lt. General Robert Baden-Powell and Walter H. Page, the American Ambassador; in 1927, Percy W. Lee invited Viscount Cave, the Lord Chancellor and Earl Jellicoe. The day after this feast, they toured the Vickers armament works.

The feast today is still an important event for making speeches and networking. The day after the feast has traditionally been for visits to local factories, to showcase Sheffield manufactures. Politicians, business leaders and dignitaries continue to be the principal guests and the Master Cutlers maintain the custom of using this occasion to advance the name of Sheffield.

References

MANUSCRIPT SOURCES
    Cutlers' Company archives:
        First account book, 1625–1790, D1/1.
        Accounts of the Master Cutlers, 1811–1889, D1/3.
        An inventory of the Cutlers' Hall, 1807, D10/1.
        Charles Belk archive, P19.

PRINTED SOURCES
    MacDonald, J. (1997) 'The Cutlers' Feast' in Binfield, C. and Hey, D. (eds.) *Mesters to Masters* (Oxford), 225–240.